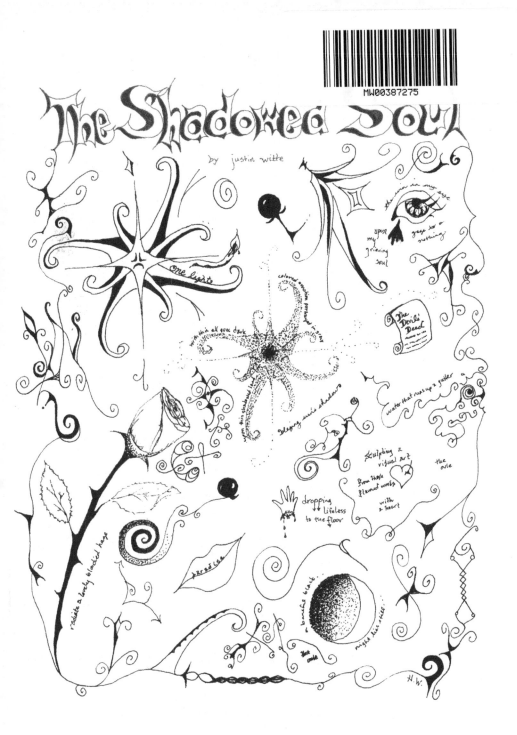

The Shadowed Soul: Poetry & Essays
by justin j. witte
fifth edition

also by justin j. witte:

A Vicious Cycle: Change for the Better

The Shadowed Soul

Poetry & Essays

fifth edition

by
justin j. witte

illustrations by
heather woods

CONTENTS

Prologue

THIS BOOK IS ABOUT OVERCOMING *mental illness through jnana yoga. Jnana in Sanskrit means mind, and the only thing that yoga means in practice. I have suffered from almost every mental illness there is with my rare organic brain disorder. I have what is called a heterotopic grey matter, which gives me the aspects of eight brain disorders without fitting one stereotype, but the point of this book is the neuroplasticity of the brain and how if we exercises our brains, and treat them right, we can heal them and get them to grow because nobody is born with an "IQ," for lack of a better term. Be that "IQ" social or intellectual. I show in my theory of the mind that, despite my unique diagenesis I am not that much different than anyone using the psychology of movies and commercials.*

I based my theory of the mind on neurological testing I had done at UCSF and I combine it with Vedanta. Vedanta is a type of Hinduism that is most similar to Buddhism and goes very well with modern science. I also like Hinduism because it addresses the paradoxes in an empirical world of relativity and duality that most modern sciences do not. Most Modern Western Sciences go by Aristotle's Law of Contradiction which states there isn't one empirical truth which will contradict another. The only Western Science that doesn't deny this is quantum physics because there is just no way around it, unless the scientist is living in denial and says "that is just its nature." Which some scientists do! Strongly disagree with Contradiction being a Law because if everything has an opposite and all perspective is relative, then we do get answers and make progress, but the paradox is there is always more questions just like the Vedic Scriptures predicted, but my true hope is that others can help others who have suffered from mental illnesses such as I have.

The poetry of this book I wrote mostly as a depressed suicidal child with a third-grade reading level. I was someone who was a functional illiterate most of my life. I remember wanting to be a writer as a child locked up in that detentionary boarding school Discovery Academy. I graduated that high school with that third-grade reading level, and I learned how to truly read at the age of 30 through the Linda Mood Bell Program, but when I wrote this poetry as a child my reading was so terrible that I had to have others do the spell check for me because of all my learning disabilities being so terrible. Even with my learning disabilities I seemed to write in a very well-structured meter.

I always wanted to help others who have suffered from suicidal depression and other mental illnesses such as I have since I have recovered and am living a happy life. I've tried to kill myself more times than I can count. A lot of it was for attention, but there were times I meant it and I just wouldn't die. I have scar on my throat that I show to others who are struggling. That scar can be very helpful sometimes for others who are suffering from the same suicidal depression I did. It blends in quite well with my razor burn so it isn't noticeable unless I show it to someone. Cutting my throat was the second time I spent a month in a psych-ward and is why I got put on SSDI. I didn't get denied for Federal Disability once. The first time I spent a month in a psych-ward was over my fourteen birthday.

I have seen doctors my whole life, and there were few really good ones, but most couldn't help me in anyway, and some, like the doctors at Discovery Academy, made my life much, much worse. I have been on almost every psychiatric drug and anticonvulsant there is, and most doctors and medications did nothing for me, but I agree with the Buddha: suffering is a universal principle of all life and selfishness is the main cause. I also *show how Sigmund Freud and Buddha come to the same conclusions too. The Buddha just offers a solution.*

I also was someone who suffered from child abuse, and I believe today that love is the only true cause of all actions. We all just have the same two problems: ignorance and understanding. I don't resent my father at all today, who was the reason I got hospitalized the first time at the age of thirteen. There is nobody to resent in my life today because this empirical world is all just cause and effect, or Karma, and I see today that the Law of Karma and the Theory of Evolution tells me the same thing: everything is constantly changing, this life is all about learning, and I either learn or I suffer. This means that nobody is born with an IQ, and we can develop our minds at any age. In each of my chapters where I talk about meditation there are mental exercise that I do daily which got me off most of my medications and has allowed me to live a happy life. I want anyone else who is suffering from mental illness to live a happy life too which is why I am sharing this story.

The Law of Karma also tells means there is only one person with the power of choice in my life: me! Not because I have it but because there is no other way to live! We are all here just for an experience and when you take the power of choice out of anyone's hand there is nobody to resent. I see everyone just doing their best and Socrates said, and there are paradoxes everywhere in this empirical world of relativity and duality such as the power of choice and determinism. That is why life have enjoyed learning all the different forms of Hinduism, especially Vedanta, and I see everything and every action as nothing but love today because we are all this energy of Loving Consciousness manifesting in this chaotic illusion called the Maya, we all just have those same two problems which leads to our troubles as I stated above: ignorance and understanding.

CHAPTER 1

The Shadowed Soul

WHY

my remorsed conscience shamed,
in soothing songs which they lack,
from bitter feelings lamed
to a loveless, grim heart of black.

by vision sweetened myth,
since before one spoke to me,
in twilight blissful with
her arms willing, open and free.

in hopeless dirgeful tears,
i acquit all i attack,
just upon sullen fears
of emotions, which i do lack!

4/03/95

THAT MIGHT BE ME I HATE

i recall his swing
as my blood flew,
screams in the night
while hatred grew.

with bottle in hand
he still must drink,
cast aside
as my heart does sink.

in silence alone
i did so weep,
with all our tears
in sorrows deep.

and upon his leave
i still do cry,
from this man
whom i wish would die.

for along these years flow swiftly by,
his thought in mind
will gently pry.

so thinking of him
others do see,
him in this picture of only me.

a downward fall I seem to concede,
with all this Rage
my soul does bleed!

for within this life's unlawful fate,
i might just be
that man i hate.

05/18/94

THE ROCKIES IN FALL

these thrilling hills so inspire
loving dreams of young hearts desire,
of goldish-red of beautied death
are calming my spirits with each breath.

ah for this dew of morning air
thrills me with love and sights so fair,
while joys of such a sweetened day
just from this merriment of my stay.

reaching the peak in the sky
the sun urges from my heart a sigh,
pondering life with meaning now
as the soothing winds caress my brow.

these songs of the birds passing call
i gaze to the thrilling his in fall,
with love in thoughts of Artemis
settles my soul in such golden bliss.

9/30/94

INNOCENT DREAMS

just with in the obscure schemes
of moments where i weave in and out
to disembodied soul,
clutter my grim sights insane,
while each wish will slowly disperse
to colored emotions portrayed in gray.

all my worries fall from love
to pity of the rich man's pocket,
yet the think of me so sick
with concerns in shamed distain,
as cold rays of bitter sunshine
show their addictions so far from their dreams.

these yearnings will enhance urges
of times where i danced from the trees,
where i imagined all bliss,
and took breaths to sooth my pain,
yet my heart has been deflowered
so i've lost the airy hopes of a child.

9/05/95

LET ME BE

let me be! just let me be!
beating this fever down on me!
let marrow fall to sooth pain,
don't veer my simple dreams insane!

let me be! just let me be!
under God's reign i'm still not free!
i just wish to be in peace,
let my Lord's ancient hymns decease!

let me be! just let me be!
fade Apollo to dusk at sea.
set spirits free of law's might,
and let night's vision hold delight.

8/01/95

A DREAM OF OPHELIA

throughout this darksome sky these violent
dim colors cast the moon's lonely tint;
which by means of dusky gold beams
leaves divine thoughts in vivid dreams,
so beatific are golden yearnings,
forth from moonlight, in blissful burnings.

vivid peeks within elate horizon
just in front of this so violet sun;
which kisses one in such a haze
of fervor in stunning blaze,
her decorum does worship implore,
with such consent, felt never before.

charming and lustful is this nepenthe
i've never been with my spirits free;
free upon this one so divine
in misty dew and flavored wine,
while emotions such loving madness,
she does vanish, in dreamy sadness.

blissful was milieu now such remorseful
dreams upon thought of a loving soul;
i progress to where she was most
to reveal not even her ghost,
such feverish thought languid moping,
as i'm humbled, in weary hoping.

4/09/95

AN ODE TO POE

i see this one i know so well
within these fiery pits of hell,
for his pen in flawless rhyme
holds my spirit in wicked time.

each word of fear can make me weep
unto a fearful purple deep,
while each one of my feelings scream
in thoughts of every vivid dream.

as dark dreams feed all my fright
moving us closer in this night,
for this man i admire so
is one such Edgar Allen Poe.

10/05/94

WHAT I'M LOOKING FOR

i'm here sitting in thought alone,
so far away from the lands i've known,
oblique thoughts of mine stray so far;
as i cast my wish to one dim star.

i do explore the thoughts of fear,
in the sorrow of each salty tear,
without the dreams of one dull hope,
i'm left here with my soul to grope.

O God wher'er your spirit be,
thru the devil's hills or deep blue sea,
divine peace of your grace shall soar,
and bestow what this heart yearns for.

2/13/95

A DOVE

beautied ink sculpts an art
with flavored words from my heart,
while dreams in mist suspended,
stir worries on my brow,
of yearnings for her love now
is no such harm intended.

Godly sign of the dove
chaste upon clouds high above—
one hoe holds my gratitude.
this zeal of her won't cease,
yet paltry is sign of peace
for my heart she does elude.

unto these tears i weep
in troubled gray tint so deep,
makes airy my heart cower.
uncouth in a charmed scheme,
is figment just sift of dream
and palm from love meant sour?

only to feel heart's beat
such vivid dreams won't deplete—
shame felt from this confession,
which leaves thoughts just to burn,
as fallen hopes with concern
scream numb thrills of depression!

decree to one i miss
in chilling pit of abyss—
comes all my frayed emotion,
which peaks where sun does dance,
while dusky blur will enhance
all my hymns of devotion.

8/07/95

A LITTLE VOICE

through the trees, i make my way,
while all such thoughts go astray,
from my heart a whisper cold,
depth of dreams have been untold.

in these voices, is unto ends,
for in my sight a nymph attends,
while he brings these shadows deep,
am i 'wake or just asleep?

is this moon, the way it gleams,
just my doubts from out my dreams?
this sprite shows a fevered bliss,
which veers my mind to madness.

tint of gray, hides all my fear,
it can't tell what will appear,
'bout this hell of bewitched sight,
is one who stalks me tonight.

i do hide, with hope to live,
as a sound holds me captive,
that sound of each crushing leaf,
as fright make me feel grief.

it's that sound, i do not doubt,
i can hear it all about,
i'm just crouching down with fear,
then they start to disappear.

through the woods, i softly creep
i try not to fall asleep,
as this voice in troubled ear,
back in thought is does appear.

7/26/95

ONLY MAN

a bomb flashes a strobe of violence
in a wave bringing our vivid fate,
coming just to burn all unto silence,
sweeping over with all of man's hate.

raging forth in the devil's savage might
shown in tears which each babe does cry,
abandoned in their blurred vision of fright,
calling to those dead under night's sky.

thinking of such war enriched by glory
until when we are in this fire,
for what's been told to me in great story,
has now crumbled to lame desire.

yet from this city's death not one can learn
while the devil will forever deed,
on fields of loved ones left to burn,
by this glory of man's sickened greed.

6/12/95

THE SHADOWED SOUL

i look where land and sky meets,
the soft night's chilling breeze
is scattering leaves across these streets,
through muscular forms of bare trees
comes the palish moon's guileful light,
to leave spirits blind, in pall of night.

thrown to the grown is shaded veil,
these shadows so dreadly told
in a moonlit night of horrid pale,
cause vigilance of winds so cold
just creeping through demonic land,
from where i have been, so wrongly banned.

i can feel my mind veer insane,
with my skin as cold as stone
so moribund in an echoed pain,
just holds me beneath Hades' throne
while ominous light's opaque dim,
is clenching my fate, by baneful grim.

8/17/95

CANNON BEACH

such aspirations i willingly squander
entangled in thought i carelessly ponder
as i lose myself in the sun's violet haze,
to dreamy colors my thrilling hopes gaze.

with aspirations in colorful delight
engaged by the fading reign of sunlight
the last bit of sunlight does vividly hold,
these colors of waves just crashing so bold.

the aspirations of violet vanish
by means of the silken shadow which banish
all but the stars with in this cold opaque sky,
lovingly sparkles in white of my eye.

this wondrous sight of the heaven above
fills me with evil, nobility, and love
that fears all in the darkest of sullen night,
i notice the fires rage to blind my drunk sight.

while aspirations of song paraded dance
within this blaze of fire my spirits chance
the drugged glory in music by my guitar,
just playing my dreams to every last star.

7/18/94

THE WORDS OUR PROPHET SENT

each soothing stroke of a violin,
is calming me from vengeful sin,
for music is my needed light,
leaves thoughts within dusky night;
as each shadow starts to mold
breast and hooves, which chills me cold.

such crying is for my heart's lament,
from bitter words our prophet sent,
like flowers on a god graced hill,
yet holds me in troubles still;
this means of sorrow will creep
and wake me, when i can sleep.

and with the thoughts of life alone,
will trouble hearts to vengeful moan,
rent delusions to heavens above,
and upon heights of dreaming love,
as serpents tongue will scorn
life of hell, for this i mourn.

10/03/94

A FOOL'S DREAM

i can feel a warm pleasure—
as my dreams fade and decease
in midst of this languished treasure,
i look to wrap myself in peace.

all faults i long to relieve,
for each thought will go astray,
while my sights shall only deceive
from my dull life's inert display.

yet when i dream i taste love,
as if cured by Goodfellow,
my heart is just compelled above
and trapped with hymns of a cello.

i crave that charmed taste of wine—
enhanced in shades of twilight,
for it stem a lustful divine
leaves me strung in vigored delight.

joys are filled to inspire—
for on longer can i wait,
to dance my heart between each fire
which leaves no dream left to create.

i start to fall from revel—
for such love could not repeat,
as my heart's most joyous devil
tells me all this will just deplete.

with my hopes unjust plunder,
comes this rage which will fervent—
and burn even sweetest wonder
to Hades most cruel descent.

7/18/95

JUST TO HOLD, JUST TO TOUCH

with reality of my illusions
i praise these moments i spend alone,
gazing to stars in shining delusions,
i hear one faintly whisper a moan.

looking to the setting where i had stepped
through this comforting yet rugged land,
where the mist and water so gently crept,
just over the rocky beach's sand.

within every thought of mine i ponder
i see one bringing her face to sight,
then yelling a frightful rage of thunder,
all such words showing my vicious might.

"Love" is her heart's dire timid response
which makes my spirits frightfully cringe,
for within that word there's something which haunts,
and confuses me with a gray tinge.

my spirits gather in lonesome parade
and still with all thoughts on days of yore,
so slowly they begin to blur and fade,
knowing i can take not one bit more.

yes fade, fade from impervious treasure
for this mortal heart so far from stone,
my loneliness is but sorried pleasure,
why should i roam loving land alone?

with all my emotions in hopeless prayer
i do so long in my dreams to touch,
ah to touch and hold i wishfully dare,
in all i ask would this be too much?

with this dream coming forth in colors bold
for i can feel the lovely moon's beams,
kissing me soft in white pearlish gold,
just calming me in the way it gleams.

7/01/94

22

THE DEVIL IN ME

here i stand in molding time,
which taunts me to brake free
from my heart's feverish wit,
comes all my dreams pointless rhyme,
to think of what will be
worth my soul's troubling fit.

should each man's thoughts worry me?
if they think i am crude,
or just not up to their par,
i am not able to see
all the whims of foes mood,
if my joys have strayed too far.

don't see a prophet of doom—
when your eyes shift to my
heart's most feverish hate,
that lingers about the room,
and seams to never die—
is this devil which hold my fate.

9/19/95

THE REASON TO LIVE

my spirit longs to beckon at the whim of the wind,
as i look to the east at this dawn and dusk,
just reflecting off this full lifeless land
of trees, hills, and cliffs misted in fog and snow.

aspirations of a silken purple land revile that beauty
which is only at the beginning and ending of all known to me,
for within the first breath of life is dreamt bliss of death,
as even purple dusk will yearn the blanket of night.

in that blanket is portrayed visions of real life
muttering a lustful dull of such lingering stars,
which gleamingly shows the truth of an errored folklore,
and grandly bestows meaning to each man's life.

12/09/12

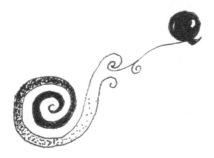

MY LAST DREAM

Ah the smell.
Just to dream the tastes
before I see what my heart
is set upon.
From the streams of Italy
I can feel the balls of meat
in my cheeks of my fevered mouth.
Then to Germany where the sausage
comes from that so
delicate and ignorant race.
With that my mind wonders to France,
where I suck the cream out of a chocolate eclaire.
All of this leaves my body so peeked!
Yet with the opening of my eyes
i look across this park of filth and dirt.
i bump my head against this crusty wooden bench.
oh well maybe tomorrows dinner.

SOUTH ROAD

as i peer through theses stalks of corn
into the berries so sweet,
i can see the hens which dream
to fly out of South Road.

on the northwest side of these hills
i yearn to be in that farm so small and fine,
which still lives in my heart
with aspirations from the days before.

through this corn i can see the willow
weeping with tremors of family life,
and points me to the forest, in dreams
of the love and victories of my foes.

these Dragons and Goblins i triumph
with my hairless hands so callused in dirt
yet all brings my loss each day
with the sun setting just forcing me home.

home, even darker than the silk of night,
which every youthful demon hides,
yet this thing which gives me life
now yearns all tortures with it.

but even my dreams are in this bitter acre of land
for it gets me to promise never to leave.
and with that oath i see men come
to chop each tree that my loving foe cowers in.

and with the falling of each tree
the hair of my hand slowly thickens,
leaving childhood dreams only to thin,
Which strengthens the tide that shipped me away.

in this sea of rock and dirt
i'm hid away in years to come.
each second seemingly takes forever,
for much happens when i think back.

each second takes forever and the days
go by with a blink, as i'm flown back home.
yet where is home? i can't see it here.
i'm on the Northwest side, but not South Road.

So with my heart's lazy desires, against all will
lie here to dream of what i had.
to all the ends the memories are cluttered with pain,
yet i even enjoy these dwelling thoughts.

but if i look back through those stalks of corn
i can see that dream i lived so full,
and i daresay not all was hell, but even joy,
for i wish i was on the Northwest side on South Road.

PLATO VS PINDAR

An ode to a common man,
whose cipher left in ancient sand,
which fade from a scholar's mind,
for flagrant is such Cronus' Time.

This God of Time cripples all,
while fire will so gently fall,
as it sparks the weeping dirge,
just robbing hope to sadly purge.

Throw each God and Hero 'side,
the basic ones have never died,
so soft his hymns gently state,
no arguer for this needed fate.

To sculpt such words upon stone,
each average soul has timeless throne,
for the sins of vivid gold,
in bludgeoned coin will future hold.

With zeal of an artful talk,
yet sadly will the scholar mock,
looks down on the folly man,
whose finding love in empty sand.

State needs of a manly lore,
each teacher I have yearning for,
yet when song and scholar fight,
the poet' one is always right.

08/10/13

MENTENSOMATOSIS

The four triangles in endless arrangements based on Forms.
the building blocks of the Earth and Heavens
the matter has always been, and so has the images of the One.
The Demiurge constructs with the intellect a living being,
these beings are the ones that study the stars,
asking questions about what comes after this life.
we die, rot in the ground, and become food for the tree.
We blossom into the flower, then develop to fruit.
We are eaten, then transmitted to the seed.
This seed is only expressed in the Dionysic hymn,
a desire within each that is created,
to only be enhanced by the grapes that are crushed,
then we die again, perpetuated in an endless circle,
which was only ended with the hemlock,
something one should never do,
yet Ananke still Unites us
with the Gods in the Tower of Kronos.

NEOLITHIC AGE

From the Neolithic age
In the langue were the w and the v interexchange
Comes an auspicious symbol
That now means to be taken as evil.
Four sides it holds
Looked at on all sides,
And now it is tilted half way to the right
Yet at the beginning of time
It meant peace, now it means war.
It was found in more than the Aryan
Circles of the North,
For all over the world before cultures
Got to know each other with the exploration
Of the free world.
In South America, India, China and more.
The symbol misunderstood and misrepresented.
The crime was against many, and even humanity itself.
The perversion of good is now
What all in the modern day take as evil.

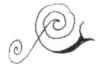

CHAPTER 2

A Glimmer of Hope

GOING IN AND OUT OF the rooms of recovery, from meeting to meeting, and treatment center to treatment center, without staying sober was the way my life was for a long time. I just had no ability to surrender. I had no ability, just like most of us, to see what I was truly thinking in anyway. It was interesting because the one thing I always did was walk back into the rooms of recovery, and I truly hated anything to do with God because of being locked up in that detentionary boarding school where I wrote all this poetry, I open the book with.

The one thing I could never give my life up to was God. I was locked up in a Discovery Academy, in the middle of Provo Utah, for three years. Discovery Academy was a one-year program which was meant for trouble privileged kids who came from disfunction, and none of their parent knew what to do with them. The only thing they did constantly was try and convert all of us to the Mormon way of life, and none of the kids came from a Mormon family except one. She was a daughter of one of the teachers who taught there.

They tried as hard as they could to convert all of us to see "their light." The fundamentalist in Utah only achieve one thing with all the kids there except one: David Jones. We also all just picked on him and called him Jesus Jones the whole time he was there. The Mormons got us all to hate God, or anything to do with God, with all our passions in our hearts. I showed how they made me feel about God in the poem *Let Me Be*. The only thing that school really made me was angrier than I already was, and worse than I already was in every single way. I was abused hard, and at the school I only perfected my Oppositional Defiance Disorder with their fundamentalist guidance.

Oppositional Defiance Disorder is a disorder kids with autism and severe Attention Deficit Hyperactivity Disorder, ADHD, are known to get, which means anyone, in any authority situation what-soever, they would stand up too! That place made my life so much worse than already I was when I was sent there. I was sent there because the psych-ward I was sent to, for my first sings of suicidal tendencies, let me go without any recommendations and my mother just did not know what to do with me. Today I see my mother had no choice, so I do not resent her in any way for it, or anything I went through as a child. If it wasn't for my mother, I doubt I would have the capacity to be as loving a person as I can be. I was just an extremely sensitive person, who still too this day takes everything personally. I was completely out of control when I was a little kid, but because of Discovery Academy, and the fundamentalists that tried to force their way of life on us all, my biggest problems when it came to the circles of recovery was God! For years after I left that place whenever I heard the word "God" anger was the only emotion I would express!

One night I was at an old Episcopal Church at Bush and Gough in San Francisco right before a meeting and I just said the words to myself: "I don't know?" It was interesting because I had never really said those words about too much of anything before. I thought about it right as I said it, and at that moment those words, "I don't know?" became my Higher Power. To say I did not know was the beginning of a true solution because once I said those words, I started to stay sober. I had a professor, who was had a PHD in theology at SFSU, years later tell me my definition of God is Socratic. It has been interesting to me that since opening my mind with those words, I have found my God in the Ancient world both Greece and India. I did a lot of soul searching in the rooms of recovery, and stayed sober, but I had a dream of doing more. I had a dream of getting off SSDI. I hated government assistance. I wanted to be somebody, not just an empty soul powerless under the hands of society who was not able to have a life because anyone with that limited income has a hard time living life to the fullest in America. I knew if I was going to amount to anything, I would need to be able to go to school, and if I went to school, I had to be able to read. All the kids I have talked to on Facebook, or in person, that went to Discovery Academy were traumatized by Discovery Academy, and most couldn't even read when they "Graduated" high school, which we all did, unless we were sent somewhere worse. I was able to graduate Discovery Academy with a third-grade reading level just like every other kid that was sent there.

It was only by pushing myself to read as much as I could, every day, with a lot of literature I could not even comprehend, that got me into college. With all of my learning disabilities, it was not just about understanding the words and the phonics but comprehending what was on the page too. My ADHD was more difficult than my dyslexia in my opinion, because once I could sound out the words, I still had a harder time focusing on the page and absorbing the content I was reading. None of the ADHD medications worked for me whatsoever, so I just had to continue to try as hard as I could to be able to understand what I was reading. It was crazy because I would be reading a book and not even be aware that I was not paying attention to the words. I'd be reading and a word would trigger a different thought, so I would be thinking of something completely different than what I was reading. I would just wake up somewhere else in the book on a different page and not even be able to remember, or processes, much of what I read if anything at all. With all of this I just pushed ahead and read as much as I possibly could every day. I read 100 pages of Kant one day when I first began reading, and the only thing I really got out of the book was the Latin phrase *a priori*: before the fact.

When I beginning to read daily, I found a great book: *Greek Thought, and the Origins of the Scientific Sprit*, by Leon Robin. I loved the way this book was written because I could comprehend phrases, and snippets of literature, which sounded poetically beautiful that Robin took from the Ancient Greek philosophers of the time. It was so creative and well-constructed. It is an older book, so the style is much different than the modern literature, but those are the authors I tend to like the most because the philosophy of the older literature is much more poetic.

This book has turned out to be my favorite book. I have read it many times, and even spending time committing pages of it to memory because I loved it so much. The Section on Heraclitus the most! It is this book that got me to memorize other phrases from books as well. Because of this book I love to find creative aphorism within them and commit them to memory, and then share them with other people when I am giving a speech at the toastmasters, a radio show, or speaking for college professors. It was also this book that inspired me to go from an accounting major to a philosophy major.

There is a line in this book which spoke to me more than any other. Robin says how Plotinus, the first of the Neoplatonists, wrote, "After rising from the Ego to the One, I now find the Ego once more, and in that Ego the Infinite One if I wish, but if I turn from it to determine my own domain and give myself the illusion of independence, then I become only a part, isolated from the Whole and am truly reduced to slavery." It sounded so cool when I read it, and it took me a little while to truly understand all of it, but what that saying means is: I go from myself up to God, and in myself I find God, and God finds Himself in me. I am One and identical with God if I have the clarity to see who I truly am and depend on God completely, but if I turn away from God, to get some type of self-independence, which I might think would make me special and unique, then I have done the wrong thing. Breaking away from God makes it that I have lost who I truly am. When I take myself as any different, unique, or independent from God, instead of being One with God, and relying on God completely, is where all my trouble lie. Relying on God completely is what I am meant to do. Being true and special is to be One with God and taking God and Everything! To be One with God, is to be a God, which is identity-in-difference. The Neoplatonists were qualified-nondualists, AKA identity-in-difference, and Neoplatonists and Vedanta, which is my spiritual practice today, have lots in common. Vedanta is just a religion practiced in the modern day of India, but what they practice is: we are all One with God and God is Everything.

It was those words which spoke to me so clearly. Even when I did not completely comprehend them, they just sounded so beautiful and pulled me right in. What these creative words did for me was make me want to seek the truth! Even when I did not understand them completely, I enjoyed spending my time doing my best to figure them out. I just got a mystical feeling form them, and they pulled me in. It was this mystical feeling which made me do research on Neoplatonism. It was that research that made me a Neoplatonist and convinced me Plato was my prophet in the West. Especially because so many of the conclusions I came to on my own were already in the Platonic and Neoplatonic texts. This goes with Plato saying how the soul has always existed; therefore, the soul has already seen everything: Anamnesis, which are numerical truths exist within us all.

If any of us want the answers to anything, just look within. Not just Anamnesis but Platonic Forms, which are the truths that makes up everything in this empirical universe, are within us all. This is why we are all fallen Gods trapped in human flesh. All the research I have done has shown me this because I am always coming across other's writing which reveals others have already come to my conclusions as well. My conclusions, which I thought were original, have already been revealed by all the other souls in history. The revelations are just universal truths within all of us. These are the platonic concepts of Forms and Anamnesis.

Because I was reading so much, once I got an iPhone, I always went to iBook's in order to download more books. They had a lot of books with expired copy writes for free there. This is where I found the book *An Essay on the Beautiful*, by Plotinus, which has been translated by Thomas Taylor and John M. Watkins.

There was also another book I read in my English 1B class in college at Community College of San Francisco, which had to be the best-written fiction book of the 20th Century in my opinion. That book was *Invisible Man* by Ralph Ellison. This book spoke to me clearly as well, so I related them both to my life, and I saw the truths in myself from a book, which was meant for an African American audience: *Invisible Man*, and I united it with the Platonic truths in *An Essay of the Beautiful*. Both these books were protreptic to me.

The etymology of this word in Latin comes from the word protepticus, which means something that is encouraging. In Greek the word would be protreptikos, which comes from another word protrepein. Protrepein in Greek means to turn forward and urge on. Protreptic in English describes an utterance, or a speech, that is designed to instruct and persuade. A moral instruction is what I would call both *An Essay on the Beautiful* and *Invisible Man*. It is writers like these, Plotinus and Ralph Ellison, that got me to see my true nature, let go of the past, and continue to strive for the better.

Plotinus teaches that the Soul is innately good, and it is in the search for truth that its goodness is revealed. In *Invisible Man*, Ellison writes about an African American in the South during segregation who is struggling to find purpose and the goodness within himself. The Invisible Man's mistake throughout the book is he is in a constant conflict with himself. What he is conflicted about is his self-worth. He constantly tries to get self-worth through the approval of others. I am not African American, but anyone should be able to relate to seeking approval from others. I my chapters on depression, anxiety, psychosis I show how too much of what we all come to think about ourselves and how we all identify, is what we think others think of us when none of us can even prove others have minds let alone what they are thinking. From what I have seen, everyone cares too much what they think the people they meet in the world think about them. This self-identity and struggle is something all humans go through and is what the ridiculous theory of race is based on. The approval from others is what caused most of my problems as a child as well. That is what my Oppositional Defiance Disorder was about. I could not get any positive attention and approval growing up, but I was extremely good at negative attention. Just like everyone else, my adolescent shaped the early years of my adult life.

In the *Invisible Man*, when the Invisible Man gets to the goal of finding out who he truly is, then he is free and no longer depends upon other people to prove he is a good and worthy person. For a large part of my life, I was in as much fear as the Invisible Man. When I finally was able to have a purpose and self-worth, I was able to let most of the fear in my life go. That fear was what was controlling me, so when I let the fear go, I was able to educate myself and started on the road to a solution and happiness. Letting go of fear, and a self-identity based on the imagination of others, was Invisible Man's solution as well.

There's education in the writing of Plotinus too. Plotinus writes, "Thus proceeding in the right way of Beauty he will first ascend into the region of Intellect, contemplating every fair species, the Beauty of which he will perceive to be no other than Ideas themselves; for all things are beautiful by the supervening irradiations of these, because they are offspring and essence of Intellect." This tells how the soul is innately good, and the way to have that realization is to use the Intellect within us all to access and see that goodness. We use this Intellect to see the answers within us all. This is for everyone. Everyone at their core is a God in themselves. We are all worthy, and there is a loving purpose for all of us. We just need to look inward to find all the answers.

To be able to see the truth is the main point of anyone's life in my opinion. The only thing that stands in anyone's way is their perception. The Beautiful is All and creates All, for this is what

Plotinus is stating. "Supervening irradiations," means to shine our goodness through. Shining our goodness through is the Intellect within ourselves revealing the answers. We are all meant to expose ourselves to the answer; not to expose ourselves to the thoughts of others like I did and the Invisible Man did, but to looking within and seeing the Intellectual Principle that Plotinus writes about in the *Enneads*. It is the Intellectual Principle which leads to the One, the Beautiful, and the Good. Those are the only three words which can describe our Maker according to Plato because there are no other words which are just for God. To Plato God is ineffable, so veg words of Perfection is all anyone can say about God! Too Simple and Perfect for words!

It is this search for who he is that makes the mind of the Invisible Man so cloudy at the beginning. In the first chapter he ends with a speech that is quite amazing and ardent. He first gets beaten to the ground, then he picks himself up and puts forth wonderful words that dictate his goals with blood dripping down his neck and in his throat. It starts out, "We of the younger generation extol the wisdom of that great leader and educator." These words here give the premise for his goal throughout the book. That goal is to seek an education. Like Plotinus he knows it is his Intellect that is the objective of his happiness. Invisible Man is intelligent, and he exposes this in each one of his speeches. His flaw is that he is looking for the approval of people whose disposition is to look down upon him for the color of his skin. He is looking for white men's approval in the South. This is nothing but insanity because none of them will ever give it to him because he is African American.

As I stated, I am a white man, but I constantly made the mistake of basing who I was on what others were thinking of me too. I have noticed this because just like Invisible Man, I had a way with words too, yet my gift with words was more about judgement. I could always see what was wrong with people and cut them down, but it was nothing but a sense of inferiority that I was blind to. It was my childhood which encouraged this behavior in me. It was my father, and then it was perfected with the trauma of Discovery Academy, which perfected this skill! This "skill" was nothing but a defense mechanism and was the cause of all of my difficulties in my life for a very long time. This fear of what my family thought, lead to the fear of what the rest of the world thought, especially those kids at Discovery Academy, who were already angry too! That all spun into anger and chaos for years! It was this anger and chaos that got me to try and kill myself me more times than I can count! This fear and anger got me to get in fights every night for a year straight in San Francisco and I did not even win one! This fear and anger got me to get arrested over and over. This fear and anger got me to use every drug there was! This fear and anger got me in and out of every psych ward in San Francisco more times than I can possibly imagine! It was only to try and find the answers, find out who I truly am, and what I truly "Do Not Know" that got me to the goal of turning my life around. Turning his life around is what Invisible Man does too! But, Invisible Man is seeking approval from everyone which means he is consumed with what others are thinking of him too! This constant seeking of approval leads to all the conflict in Invisible Man's life. Invisible Man is extremely talented. He has an amazing talent of speech most could never even dream of having, yet throughout the book he is in a struggle and limiting himself because he holds himself to what others think of him! It is a limit he puts on himself, just like I did, and just we all do at one time in our lives when it comes to our identity and how we define ourselves! Everywhere in my life I have seen how we all do this to varying degrees. I only know this because I have never met anyone I could not make angry with what I said to them. When lots of these people I did not even know or would never see again! Why would anyone care what a crazy little angry stranger had to say to them, but one night when I was arrested in a drunk tank, I had everyone in all the other cells screaming at me! Why would the other prisoners care, and why would the cops care? It made no sense to care what a crazy angry drunk person was saying in a different cell, but all of humanity struggles with what we think others think of us because we survive in tribes, groups, cities, and societies! We survive together, so we all struggle with this imaginary identity, and because the *Invisible Man* is so well written anyone should be able to relate to this struggle of identity if they can put their own ignorance and judgements aside on race and just look at the words of a beautifully written book!

There were always those ones who would scream at me, "I don't care what you think!" That is when I would tell them: the only ones they are fooling are themselves. If someone does not care what another thinks, there is no need to tell them they do not care because if you tell someone you do not care, you are trying to prove a point, and if you are trying to prove a point you are trying to convince someone else of something. If you are trying to convince someone of something, you obviously care what they think! It is all a defense mechanism. A defense mechanism was my problem too, and so many of our problems no matter what the color of our skin. We can all relate to getting some type of sense of self on how we compare to others, which is nothing but being consumed with what they think of us because we grow up in these family, tribes, cities and societies and we all survive together. I was constantly trying to get approval from others, and at the same time trying to prove to the world I did not care what they thought. It was the fact I so desperately did care that had driven me crazy too just like Inviable Man, but it was this fear of people got me to lash out at all the people around me and ruin my life for years!

At the end of *Invisible Man's* speech in the first chapter, he accidently utters the word "equality." This word sends the white people almost into apoplexy, for they are all appalled that a Negro in the South during segregation would be trying to achieve equality. It is this misspoken word that tells what he is truly looking for. To be loved and appreciated and taken to be just as worth as anyone else is the main desire in anyone's life if they can acknowledge it or not.

I remember being young in grade school, and it was extremely difficult for me. Being a functional illiterate most of my adult life, it was these learning disorders that dominated both my purpose and existence. I remember being asked to read out loud in Holly Trinity, which was the name of my grade school, and all of the terror that came with that. I was terrified because it all seemed so easy to the rest of the class. I felt horrible because the rest of them could seem to read so easily. It was the fear that others could do something that my brain was not permitted to do at the time. It was not that I did not want to learn. I did. I just did not have the ability to comprehend basic words that were on the page in front of me, and none of the teacher new how to help me either with my complex brain. I could not process any of the words with my Dyslexia. I could not even sound too many of the words our or comprehend them once I did. I saw all the other kids do it and automatically I felt less than, and one of the words that I longed for in school was this "equality." Or just belonging. Which is what the Invisible Man wants too. I just wanted this love and acceptance that we are all craving and misunderstanding. This Love of the One which we all truly are!

My father had his Doctorate in Organic Chemistry, and for his only son to be so terrible in school was the shame of the household. My father drilled it into my head how worthless I was because of it. My father abused me severely in lots of ways which is expressed in the poetry I open the book with, and the only thing my father could say to me when I asked him if there was anything he ever regretted about all the abuse was after he had left the house was, "I didn't make you work harder because where you are in school right now." With those words I snapped. This is what the thoughts he had of me in his mind did to me! Those thoughts of worthlessness turned out to be the thoughts which perpetuated my cycle of insanity for years. The fear of what other people thought of me was what saturated my brain all throughout my early life. Then when I went from that psych-ward as a child to Discovery Academy my life was chaos for years because of the fear of people! This fear did not end until I used my intellect to redirect all the energy I had into finding a way to get an education. An education I always wanted.

I have always wanted to learn; in fact, I found a lot of things fascinating that most people would probably take as boring, like math and physics. My hero was Einstein as a little kid, for he suffered from dyslexia as well, and some even speculated he was on the autism spectrum like me. Einstein did terrible in school and as a child had a nervous breakdown himself, but Einstein did not let it stop him. His brain was even stolen, and it kept at the Mutter Museum, and one of the things it shows is that it is a tiny bit smaller than the average brain, but Einstein went to a special school as a child, and they taught him to read a different way. It was based on picturing images when he read things.

I learned how to read as an adult at the age of 30 at a program called Linda Mood Bell. Linda Mood Bell functions off of picturing what one reads too, just like the how Einstein learned how to read. I would read a paragraph, then tell the tutor exactly what was in my mind. I would do this with as much detail as possible, even picture and describe things that were not in the text. Each paragraph was a different painting, and this was to train one's brain to comprehend the words on the page.

I am different in lots of ways because of my brain, and one of the ways I am different is I do not think in pictures at all. I think in words. This is why what Linda Mood Bell did for me was a bit different with reading the comprehension. A was also on medication at the time I took their program which retarded my thinking. Those medications are necessary when someone is struggle with psychosis and mania, like I did, but even with those medications the Linda Mood Bell program still drilled into my head was the phonics of the English language in an amazing way. I have read every day since then, and a lot of what I read was way above my reading level at the time I was trying, like Immanuel Kant, but this dedication and desire to learn, combined with the Linda Mood Bell program, got me to be able to read, and today I can read authors most people have no ability too. I just pushed myself as hard as I could because

I wanted to learn, and I wanted most of all to be off of SSDI. It was not just the sciences I found interesting, for one of the dreams I had as a child was to be a writer. That is what the poems I opened the book with were all about.

When I was at Discovery Academy is when I wrote most of the poems I opened this book with. I told myself I wanted to be a writer someday when I was locked up there. I wanted to put my ideas on paper and try and communicate a good message to other people. I promised Heather Woods, the girl who drew the cover of that book, I would publish those poems with that cover someday when I left.

It was when I finally got sober with those words "I don't know" that people would always thank me when I shared from the floor in different 12 step meetings. They do not do that too often for anyone, but lots of people truly loved what I had to say once I started living in the solution. Like Invisible Man, I have always had a talent for words like I said, but I was terrified, and I could not see that it was only fear that was controlling me. I could not acknowledge I was just basing my sense of self on what the others thought of me, just like Invisible Man did, just like we all do. We all want to be important. Ralph Waldo Emerson, not the Emerson in this book: *Invisible Man*, but the one history is familiar with, said it best, "The most basic human desire is a need of importance." That is all racism truly is. Racism is nothing but how important one person is compared to how important another person is based on something as artificial as the amount of vitamin D in the skin, which is all the color of anyone's skin is!

The amazing thing is that 99.9% of all human DNA is identical, so genetically and even behaviorally speaking, race does not even exist! The theory of race is engrained in the human psyche to seek some type of meaning and importance in our lives. We all have that insanity of worrying about the world's thinking just like the Invisible Man, and if you ask most people today, they tell you they believe in "race" when it does not even exist! This was Invisible Man; this was me. I was not discriminated with race, but I had a huge fear of people, just like Invisible Man, just like we all do, and just like Invisible Man and everyone else we all believe things that are not true! Having misbeliefs of the Empirical world and where we all fit into the society around us is an insanity all humanity struggles with! Being wrong about the empirical world and having misjudgments is a difficulty we all suffer from! Ignorance is insanity as well when it is coupled with the pride of humanity! We just need to see that to be great is in all our natures, just like Plotinus writes. We are all identical with God! We are a piece of him, and when we take ourselves as separate is when we truly suffer!

To search for my true Platonic nature is what got me to increase my reading comprehension. Linda Mood Bell was a great program for me because it got me to open the door to better reading skills. It is an amazing program that is about the neuroplasticity of the human brain and increasing oxygen flow to parts of the brain which are underdeveloped with people with learning disabilities like I have. I wish anyone with ADD, ADHD, dyslexia or autism could take it, but it was my own desire to know more and be a writer that got me to push myself as hard as I could. I read every single day, and I make sure I do not miss a day!

Since I have been reading so much, I have been able to see how I love the way Plotinus writes *An Essay on the Beautiful.* "If, in this case, every lover of truth will only study a language for the purpose of procuring the wisdom it contains and will doubtless wish to make his native language the vehicle of it to others." This line expresses the purpose of why anyone would want to be a writer of philosophy. To convince people not only of what the writer has been through, but to show a solution and truth that others can apply to their lives is the purpose of any philosophical writer. This is why one would strive for a career in writing and philosophy. I needed to learn how to read, and I needed to learn how to write, and learning is the only thing which has gotten me out of my disorders and into society instead of an endless cycle of psych wards and jail cells. It is this goal of learning, and being able to read and go to college, that got me to happiness. I was able to get my BA in philosophy and have taken several graduate courses as well. I have only paused to make more money and follow a career in law instead. I still work on learning every day, and to be a philosopher means you need to read more than any other major there is, which I do! It is not just simple text as well, but the most difficult of any text. The hardest reading there is, is in philosophy, and I have done it, and I love it! And Linda Mood Bell made all the difference!

Invisible Man, after the Bloody Battle Royal in the first chapter, leaves with the gift of pursuing an education. One of the gentlemen who is in charge of his fate is an older white man called Emerson. Emerson says to Invisible Man, "Ambition is a wonderful force, but sometimes it can be blind." This statement is the key to the Invisible Man's suffering throughout the book. He wants to be important so badly, that he cannot see his true motivation. His motivation is fear. He does not pursue his education for the fact of pure knowledge. Invisible Man is very intelligent, yet having his own intellect is not enough for him. It is his battle, and it is a battle he cannot win. Instead of finding the Beauty in his Soul, for the fact of his Intellect, he is left chasing after something that he will never get: the approval of others.

I myself am guilty of a lot of the same character defects that Invisible Man displays. I was given an IQ test as a kid because they thought I was so stupid, yet I scored a 124 which is in the top 5%. I have pages of books in my head just from listening to them before I could read. I have people's bank account numbers and social security numbers in my head from just hearing people say it once. All from just listening to them. Hearing things was the only way I could memorize things, and knowing I have this talent is not enough. I have an ego. My ego tells me to show people all the time what I can do. That is why, even being a white male, I can identify with Invisible Man. This is what makes Ellison such a great writer.

When any person can relate to the story, the writer will know they have succeeded, especially when someone that the book was not even intended for can relate because this book was written for the African American plight, but even as a privileged white person, I could relate. It is like the African American feminist Maya Angelo said, "We are more alike than unalike. Nothing human can be alien to me." Approval is a disgusting word, for it can blind my actions just like the ambitions of Invisible Man, just like the actions of all of us. Approval is based on attention. When all I seek is attention, I know I am living in fear. Fear is the enemy of the truth, and I have seen every person in my life seek this in some way because of our humanity and our surviving together.

Plotinus writes about a black blanket of fog that shadows the truth as well. "But, though the mischief arising from the study of words is prodigious, we must not consider it as the only cause of darkening the splendours of Truth, and obstructing the free diffusion of her light." With this passage it tells there are those who do not speak the truth, and even write words that are based in error. It is up to the Soul to see the truth. For perception is enhanced and clarified only through trial and error. To make the judgment of what one would want to believe in. When someone speaks with words of anger and vitriol, it is up to another to see if it does hold true for them. When Plotinus argues the nature of the Soul to be Good, that tells me that if I look with persistence, I will see the truth. That truth will be what brings happiness and freedom.

It is also in a cloud of lies that a man called Brother Jack tries to use the talents of Invisible Man, so he can get his way. Brother Jack asks the Invisible Man, "How would you like to be the next Booker T. Washington?" Booker T. Washington was a African American who lived in America in the South from April 5th 1856 to November 14th 1915. He was a true person of American history who bowed down to the white establishment in the South for his own benefit. The white people wanted this because Booker T. Washington was able to get the other African Americans to be more subservient to the white power. It is in these words of deceit that Brother Jack is trying to entice Invisible Man with the reward of recognition that he has been looking for. Brother Jack is offering him what he's always wanted, which is status and recognition. Yet he is doing it, not for the welfare of Invisible Man, but so he will have more control over other African Americans. This is a falsehood, and it is the same "darkening of the truth" that Plotinus writes about.

I have had others tell me to live in ways that I came to see as fake as well. People in recovery have told me that "I can't think my way into right acting, I can only act my way into right thinking." Or "Why is not a spiritual question." This seemed to be nothing but a justification of their ignorance to me. It was a brainwashing for one's actions. I understand what they mean by this. It tells me that I am to do what is right, and not always trust my thinking. When I do what is right, that will make me happy. To live in a solution, is what the truth is all about.

The problem with "I cannot think my way into right acting, I can only act my way into right thinking" is all action is based in thought, which I prove in *The Power of Inaction*. When I have clarity of mind and see all my thoughts clearly, I can see I have conflicting thoughts and emotions, just like *Invisible Man*. The thoughts and emotions can be in conflict, but only with clarity of our minds do any of us take the right action. This is the most powerful aspect of Ellison's writing. Ellison writes about a dichotomy in everything that Invisible Man experienced. Invisible Man goes from triumph to tragedy all in one sentence, which shows a true artist. I have those thoughts that I am either going to pass all my classes with honors and win the Nobel Prize, or I will not amount to anything! This is the main reason I related to Invisible Man so much. It is a powerful lesson to learn. That lesson is that the right "choices" are up to me and my Soul, which has been blessed with Beauty according to Plato. To see the truth and make the right choice about anything is a good purpose.

When it comes to "Why is not a spiritual question" they are just saying they don't have the answer. So, then they are telling you because they can't figure it out, don't ask the question. That in itself only perpetuates the ignorance. If we say you can never ask a question and the answer comes along, no one would be able to recognize the answer. Just say the words "I Don't Know?" and then, if the answer comes you can be open to that solution and truth.

It is with this keen sight of truth that Plotinus writes, "Let us quit the study of particulars, for that which is general and comprehensive, and through this learn to see and recognize whatever exists." This shows the truth available to all! If any of us can put aside all judgment, and take a comprehensive look at everything, we will find any answers we need. Misery is unlocked with the ability to see and accept what is true. All solutions are within everyone's grasp, and as long as we all try, the answers will become apparent to all of us. Satisfaction is that life is about learning, and "responsibility rests upon recognition" like Professor Bell would always say in my English 1B class at CCSF. Getting answers is the essence of what Plotinus means when he says the Soul is Beautiful. It is in the Beauty where the answers lie.

The truth is revealed to Invisible Man at the end as well, for he asks himself "Why should an old slave use a phrase as, this and this or this has made me more human, as I did in my speech?" This is the truth that Invisible Man comes to recognize at the end, and it is a question which is all about "why." He is Human, and he does not need to rely on the validation of a third party to be his truth. Every error he made throughout the book led him to the point of finding his self-worth. He is worth enough for being who he is. He has a Soul just like Plotinus and any other white man. He is able to see the truth just like we all can. The truth was there for him at the end because he kept looking, and when he found out who he truly was he found the happiness in himself.

It is in the words: "I don't know" that I define my higher power. I do believe all of my answers are within me, and to continue to look each and every day with meditation. All of the answers for the universe are within us all. As long as we can learn and look for the truth, we can be happy, but admitting we do not know, and always being able to search for another answer is where one finds happiness. Anyone can be happy when they comprehend reality. Finding the truth in every experience, and when we learn from any situation, no matter what the tragedy or reward, using the words "I don't know" is what led me to my rewards! I am arguing it will for you too in this book, and all our brains have a neuroplasticity that needs to grow and develop throughout all our lives.

This is what got me into the different forms of Hinduism because it goes every well with modern science and is all about seeking the truth. Gandhi said, "I am a passionate seeker of the truth which is just another name for God." It is in the seeking of the truth that all of the answers to life will be found. We can always be grateful as long as we learn from the struggles we go through. I have struggled with lots of things, not only learning disabilities, but to have each struggle is an experience and an opportunity to grow. This book that I have written is about the neuroplasticity of the human brain and how similar we all are. How none of us are born with an IQ and we can all get our brains to develop throughout our lives at any age. The effort I put in is a daily effort to overcome my "eight" brain disorders. I also don't fit one stereotype, but I show how similar I am to everyone else in the chapter *The Power of Inaction*, so if anyone is struggling, my hope is they can overcome their difficulties by exercising and training their mind too just like the Linda Mood Bell program is all about.

I, and everyone else, can only learn through experience. Like in *An Essay on the Beautiful* and *Invisible Man* we can find the truth as long as we will always question and never give up looking into ourselves and letting the light of our Souls shine through. Having the ability to read such reflective and protreptic words of writers such as these was necessary for me, so thank you Linda Mood Bell. Linda Mood Bell made it so I was able to get an education. Reading is a wonderful tool that is necessary for learning the lessons in these two amazing books: *An Essay on the Beautiful* and *Invisible Man*, and the only secret to life there is for any of us is the need to be willing to learn!

CHAPTER 3

Pseudo-Laws and Pseudo-Morals

THOMAS AQUINAS WRITES IN *Law, Question 90 of the Essence of Law,* that Aristotle said, "the intention of the lawgiver is to lead all men to virtue" (Aquinas P15), yet the only true law that leads all men to virtue is the *Law of Love,* which is defined as: "love thy God, thy neighbor, and thy enemy as thyself." All the laws of any government, or societies, are based on some form of RCBAs: Risk Cost Benefit Analysis. RCBAs are laws that have both virtues and vices. RCBAs is what I would also take the *613 Commandments* of the *Old Testament* as, as well.

Different people of a society get different benefits from the laws that are passed from those societies. For thousands of years the *613 Commandments* of the *Old Testament* where laws that helped govern any society. These *613 Commandments* still shape how our different societies function to this day such as: Thou Shal not Kill. Yet, some people do not get any benefits of laws that are passed by governing society, and some get harmed by the laws which the lawgiver creates; therefore, laws of a society, or even the *Old Testament,* are not laws according to Aristotle. This means that any other law that does not lead virtue to "all men" are pseudo-laws according to Aristotle; therefore, the laws any lawgiver creates are RCBAs Laws because they do not bring virtue to "all men."

It is a fact that not all laws lead "all men" to virtue; so, I do not see how Aquinas can truly say: "The *Old Laws* restrains the hand, and The *New Law* controls the mind" (Aquinas p26). By the *Old Law* Aquinas is writing about the *Laws of the Old Testament*, and by the *New Laws* Aquinas is talking about the *Law of the New Testament*. My whole premise of this book is that if we can understand our own mind; therefore, "control" our mind, then our hand will follow. As I prove in the following chapter, *The Power of Inaction*, the *Rgveda* says quite clearly: "When purified by rays of intelligent discrimination, then thoughts in the mind will humbly submit to wisdom," but this chapter will be proving that the only law that brings virtue to "all" is the *Law of Love*. As I will also prove using Vedanta that love is the root of all emotions anyway because God is everything; therefore, love is the root control all the actions of all life in every way no matter what. We all just suffer from two problems: ignorance and understanding. This means any actions that anyone takes that harm another, be them encouraged by laws of a society, or even of the *Old Testament*, are just based on the each of our misunderstandings of our situation. The only true evil there is, is ignorance. This also means that there is no reason to hate or be angry at anyone when we truly understand what controls us, and all our problems is just misunderstanding of the lack of knowledge, because God is everything and we are all One.

Let's first accept the premise that laws, even pseudo-laws, are based on morals. Since there is only one law that is not a pseudo-law, the *Law of Love*, then the only moral which a law can be based on is the only true emotion we all have: love. Since the only moral that there is, is love, and that by definition all pseudo-laws are not truly laws, then all the other morals men might have would be pseudo-morals; therefore, the lawgiver creates laws based on RCBAs. These RCBAs are pseudo-laws based on the lawgiver's pseudo-morals and the misunderstandings that we all have for ourselves, the empirical world (Maya), and another. This is because the lawgiver himself does not base the laws of society on love but on RCBAs, which are necessary because we are all suffering from this ignorance and misunderstanding of the empirical world (Maya) around us – even the lawgiver of a society.

Jesus threw out the *Old Laws* of the *Old Testament* in *The Sermon On The Mount*. Such an *Old Law* is: "eye for eye, tooth for tooth." "Eye for eye, tooth for tooth" is not compatible with love thy enemy as thyself. This clearly shows how the *Old Laws* do not bring virtue to "all men;" so, the *Old Laws* are pseudo-laws. If we are going to live by what Jesus preached, it would be nothing but insanity to try and reconcile laws which contradict each other; therefore, Aquinas is showing his insanity in trying to reconcile laws which are not compatible in anyway with the *Law of the New Testament*. Especially because Aquinas did not believe in paradoxes of an empirical world because he was a Peripatetic. It was also these *Old Laws* that were used to bring about the justifications of such chaos and terror as Colonialism which came to devastate out planet, and we are still living those consequences to this day.

The problem with "The *Old Law* is for ruling the hand, and the *New Law* is for controlling the mind," is all "voluntary" action is based in thought, then propelled by emotion. I prove determinism, and none of us have the power of choice and the only way for the individual to live is through free will in *The Power of Inaction*. This means that the only person who has the power of "choice" in my life is me, and the only person who has the power of choice in your life is you. Not because either of us have the power of choice, but because taking responsibility for our actions is the only true way any of us can learn and grow for the better, and the best way to take responsibility is to live by the power of "choice." We all need to be shaped by our consequences to the best possible outcome, which is to be held responsible for our actions. This means the only thing which needs to be "controlled" in any way is our own minds, and as I stated above, when the mind is "controlled," the hand will follow. These premises are proved throughout this book in the different chapters over and over as I show how similar we all are, and how all our realities are nothing but what we think and our minds are nothing but imagination.

In *The Power of Inaction*, the next chapter, I show how when we can see our minds clearly, from all angles, at any time of the day, through a daily practice of single pointed concentration meditation (Trataka), then we are able to make the "right decisions" through awareness. If someone is going to live by the only law which is truly a law, the *New Law*, is also about a peaceful mind. The only emotion that will propel someone to the right action every time is a true understanding of love and what the *New Law* truly means. This is what Jesus meant when he preached the only true law there is the *Law of Love*. This shows that the purpose of living one's life is to live only by understanding our true motives and intentions and practicing them to the best of our ability.

When people think of what they would call morals, people think of universal principles we all should live by. The only difficulty with this concept is people cannot completely agree on what is moral, or even what is virtuous. This means morals, when it comes to the individual, are relative if they are anything besides "love your God, neighbor and enemy as thyself;" therefore, these relative morals are the pseudo-morals.

Relativity itself is only an empirical concept. This is because the subjective view we all get is based on our unique standing and our unique experience in the empirical world, which is the Hindu concept of the Maya as well, yet if it be a universal truth, or a universal law, then it would be that of God, which God in Himself is not relative, but absolute, no matter how we define him. God in Himself is universal, yet the basic human existence of the physical body in the empirical world is relative. A human mind is only meant for understanding limited subjective concepts in an empirical world and will never be able to understand the universal such as God. This subjective understanding is why the pseudo-laws have been created in this empirical world (Maya) because we are all ignorant all the time.

"Thee Philosopher," which is how Aquinas refers to Aristotle, is an empiricist. In the painting drawn in *The School of Athens*, painted by Raphael, Aristotle is signaling towards the ground to show Plato where the truth is: here in this empirical or physical world (Maya). Plato, who was a rationalist, is signaling to the Heavens. For Plato the truth is rational, and in the heavens, because this empirical world is full of too many contradictions, or paradoxes, which violate logic according to Plato and any logician. This is shown over and over in modern science too, with such things a quantum physics.

Quantum physics is nothing but paradoxes: the electromagnetic effect, ghost action, and quantum gravity are all paradoxes, and if we are either in a digital world or a continuous digital world, either result would still be a paradox! So, all of those theories, or options we are left with the describe the empirical world are nothing but paradoxes! So, so much for the *Law of "Contradiction"* to explain the empirical world as Thee Philosopher did! The *Law of "Contradiction"* is what Aristotle championed and states there cannot be any such thing as an empirical truth which contradicts another empirical truth: paradoxes are not allowed, but the paradox of Modern Western science is every answer we get just leads to more and more questions, which is exactly what the *Vedic Scriptures* predicted! That is why to me the concept of the Maya is much, much better definition when it comes to what we see, taste, touch, and all else in this physical world.

Yet, I would argue that Aristotle did not have a good idea of what is truly virtuous either because he held himself, and all modern scientists, to that "fact" that empirical world would not contradict itself. I have even shown serval professors I have taken classes from who live by Aristotle's *Law of "Contradiction,"* the fact that we are nowhere near the *Theory of Everything*, and every time we get an answer in Western Science, it just leads to more and more questions. This is exactly what they predicted in Ancient India, and so far, Aristotle has been wrong about everything in the empirical world! I am doubting his conclusions on virtue as well as Aquinas's in this essay! That is the main concept of the Maya in different forms of Hinduism that I have explored: paradoxes and every answer just leads to more questions. One thing I would point out is that controlling the mind would be a rational solution just like Plato is signaling as well; so, the only true problems we all have are in our minds. The Colonialists also used Aristotle's concepts of virtue to justify slaver and the conquering and killing of natives all over the world in the name of Christ!

In the book *Greek Thought and the Origins of the Scientific Spirit*, Leon Robin writes how Aristotle believed in two types of people: slaves and non-slaves. Even in the days of Aristotle there were those who questioned how anyone could justify slavery. Robin writes how some say we justify slavery through war. Aristotle was saying it was fine for the Athenians to conquer the barbarians and subjugate them. Aristotle thought the barbarians should be slaves because of their inferiority.

Aristotle's justification for slavery was that the slave is nothing but a tool. Just like the "body is to the soul" (Robin P273), so the slave is to the master according to Aristotle. Aristotle was saying that there are "just" forms of slavery. "Like the ox, he has no reason, except what is valuable for his physical constitution, which is not even that of a free man" (Robin P273). Aristotle here is referring to a human slave being nothing more than an animal, just like the ox is. In fact, Aristotle refers to the slave is to the master just like the plow is to the ox. This was considered a moral law by Aristotle, but Aristotle contradicts himself by saying the lawgiver "brings virtue to all men." Slavery does not bring virtue to the slave, and what we have found in the modern day is all human DNA is 99.9% identical and such concepts of race are based on a difference of less than .1% of our genetics; so, there is no such thing as race. Sure, they did not know anything about DNA in Ancient Greece, but we can easily see how much alike we all are if we investigate and just get to know each other like any empiricists such as Aristotle would claim to do himself. We can all easily see race is a false construct about money and power if we just get to know each other and love them.

So, what Aristotle was using were nothing but the RCBA's. All any Peripatetic is trying to do with the validation of slavery would be to justify their own dominance in their society. Slave maters just wanted power. A want and a need is nothing but a desire, and desires are what controls all actions of all life, which means the problem of all life is understanding their desires. Slavery itself, at any time, was nothing but a justification of the dominant society's selfish desires. The Athenians had no need to understand or love anything but themselves, which is the problem of all life.

Aristotle says there are three types of government, and when used correctly, they bring virtue to its constituents: kingship, aristocratic oligarchy, and republic (Robin). The problem with his thinking is no government has ever been shown to bring virtue to "all" its constituent. Winston Churchill famously said, "Democracy is the best of the worst forms of government." Churchill meant that there are problems with every form of government, and this is because no matter which society, everyone has some problems of their selfishness and their moral relativity.

No society is completely free of this selfish conflict that we all have with each other because with all forms of life, life does not exist, because life cannot take action, without desire. This selfishness is why we fight. Instead of working with each other to find the common good, we fight! This fighting is something that even happens in the societies with each other when it comes to specific court rulings.

Roe vs. Wade is a good example of a moral relativity that causes all types of conflict in America. In the FindLaw Career Center, there is a paper that gives the specific details of *Roe vs. Wade*, and how the Supreme Court came to the conclusions that it did. FindLaw Career Center writes how the Supreme Court said that to restrict people from having abortions violates both the 9th and the 14th Amendments. The Supreme Court even goes on to overrule the Laws of the States which criminalized abortion. The ruling had to do with the right to privacy, and women being able to make that decision with their doctor in the 9th and 14th Amendments. I would argue, which I have told several Christians on Facebook through conversation, if you are a Christian, it does not matter what anyone does, even a woman who is wanting an abortion, the only thing Christ commands them to do to anyone, no matter what they do, is love them, which, in this case, these fundamentalist Christians are clearly not doing. The *Bible* also writes over and over how "the breath of life" is how we define life. So, there is relativity in the interpretations of the *Biblical Scriptures* as well.

This ruling has resulted in all kinds of conflict in America. There have been acts of violence taken out on the women, the doctors, and the clinics that facilitate the abortions. These acts of violence have to be based on pseudo-morals. It is the Christians themselves which are the perpetrators of these violent acts in America. Christians are supposed to be about the This Universal Law of *The New Testament*: The *Law of Love*, but to attack a woman for choosing to terminate a pregnancy is obviously not love, and not loving their enemy, and when they vote for people like Herschel Walker, we can all tell they don't care about abortion so much as they care about race. None of Herschel Walk's voters, who claim to care about abortion, cared that his African American fetuses had been aborted. They just were thrilled that he was pro-life so they might not lose another white baby.

These Christians have a problem with the woman that does not love their unborn and let the fetus live, yet they do not love the woman, accept her, and forgive her for any sins they think she commits by terminating her pregnancy; therefore, since neither of these acts are about love, if one has an abortion, or one judges or attacks a woman for having an abortion, they are both stuck in the pseudo-morals. Neither action is a loving outcome. *Roe vs. Wade* is an RCBA because one claims it is hurting the unborn, and the other says their freedom should not be restricted. If we restrict the freedom of a woman, we are not showing love towards her. The complications that are brought up in a woman's life with any pregnancy can be beyond what lots of us can understand without the direct experience in that financial situation with those medical conditions. To not allow each mother their own rights over their own bodies is to not show love for that mother, and if a mother is not able to provide a loving life for a new born, that is not love for the new born child, so the most loving thing any of us can do is allow a woman to have "control" over her own body.

Another law that has to do with pseudo-morals is *Michigan vs. EPA*. In *Michigan vs. EPA*, the Supreme Court ruled based on RCBA. *Michigan vs. EPA* was about greenhouse gas emissions and how they pollute the environment and cause people harm. The *Harvard Law Review* writes a perfect description of this ruling, and it was Supreme

Court Justice Antonin Scalia who writes the majority opinion.

Harvard Law Review writes how Scalia said in the majority opinion that the restrictions that the EPA puts on power plant emissions have to be: "appropriate and necessary." The EPA wanted to restrict greenhouse gasses that came out of power plants to protect both people and the environment. It was the States that took the EPA to court because the States said that the restrictions that the EPA were putting on the power plants were too costly. The States wanted to save billions of dollars at the expense of the health of the citizens and the environment. Scalia agreed with the States writing the EPA was not "appropriate and neces- sary" with its restrictions that it imposed at the cost of the States. This ruling either way would either cost more money, or it would pollute the environment, which is an RCBA in either circumstantial outcome.

If someone would ask Scalia: was he a moral man? Scalia would say that he was. He would say that he is moral even though Scalia is putting a price on the poor people's heads that are living around these power plants because the people who are most affected by pollution are poor people. It has to do with where these people's living spaces are. This shows that even when people are being selfish or making a law at the expense of people's health in a society, they still think they are being moral because most people never want to do the loving thing of questioning their own thinking and conclusions that they come to. It is amazing to me that it is these Southern America States that continually get devastated by these hurricanes. These Southern Christians just have too much of what they call the greatest of all sins in their doctrine because none of them want to admit Global Warming. This is why pride is the greatest of all sins because pride tells us we are right when we are wrong, and it is the love of money above the environment and health of the people that is the motivation of Scalia's majority opinion.

Scalia put the love of money above the love of thy neighbor, and either ruling would have been at either the expense of the State or the health of the American Citizens, and Scalia should have known that in *Timothy 6:10* it clearly states that "the love of money is the cause of all calamities. Some people, eager for money, have wandered from their faith and pierced themselves with many griefs," which these fossil fuel consumptions, and the love of money, is the main driving factor of global warming. These companies want the money produced by the sales of fossil fuels, and the rest of us have our selfish desires being fulfilled when it produces electricity and the power for our cars and transportation.

Another court case that showed that not everyone loves their neighbor and their enemy, is *Matal vs. Tam. Matal vs. Tam* is about the contrast between hate speech and free speech. Supreme Court Justice Alito wrote the majority opinion for *Matal vs. Tam*. The majority opinion states the First Amendment does not allow hate speech. Alito writes about how the First Amendment uses the word "persons," and this goes to the protection of any racial minority. Alito was stating that hate speech is not free speech.

Matal vs. Tam ruled quite contrary to the 2016 election and what Donald Trump ran on. Trump clearly ran on ostracizing minorities, specifically Muslims. This clearly goes against the ruling of *Matal vs. Tam*, but it did not stop the supporters of Donald Trump and the message he ran on. Trump, when he came into office, tried to get a Muslim ban for certain countries based on his bigotry, and his justification for that was RCBA because he was stating that terrorists are from the Muslim countries. This was not true, but it was still an RCBA because the people who elected Trump took the Muslims as a threat to their country. Trump was the lawgiver in this case. The Supreme Court finally ruled in favor of the Muslim ban and stated restricting immigrants is within the executive power. They also said it was not discriminatory when Trump clearly stated over and over what he was doing. It was the Christians of America who wanted this Law, which clearly is not love thy neighbor, and if the Christians took Muslims as their enemies, all they should do is love them if they are going to live up to what Jesus preached to them to do.

The reason for *Roe vs. Wade, Michigan vs. EPA,* and *Matal vs. Tam* had to do with the RCBA is that there is a risk involved with each one of these decisions against the benefits people would get out of enacting them. An RCBA is saying, according to K. S. Shrader-Frechette in *The Conceptual Risk of Risk Assessment*, that we weigh the pros and cons of each decision and say what is right for society and ourselves. Shrader-Frechette says we do not do this with personal decisions, but Shrader-Frechette is wrong. We do, do this with personal decisions.

Shrader-Frechette says there is no way for a human to sit and calculate in each decision what is RCBA, but people are constantly thinking to themselves before they take an action: "which action should I take?" Even if people do not stop and ponder that question, they are still going to be taking the action which their mind tells them is the best decision for that moment. They take that action of what they think will benefit them the most and harm them the least. We all do this. This is what Socrates meant when he said, "The passionate man and the vicious man are men who do not know their own good, who have not perceived the essence of man in themselves: No one is wicked willingly. Reciprocally, the virtues are branches of knowledge; to know is to do." (Robin p139). This means that when we truly see and understand what is virtuous, and see our minds clearly, we take the right action. We all just have the same two problems: ignorance and understanding. Why does any take any action besides what they think is best in the moment. Sure, it may be dishonest, or mean, or some other misgiving, but we all take what we think is best in that very moment, so we all have the same two issues: ignorance and understanding. This is why there is usually some form of pro and con in each action we take in this empirical illusion (Maya); so, most actions are nothing but RCBA for the average person. But with these decisions, what does it mean to make the right decision? What is love, and how can people live by that?

The most universal definition of love I have come up with would be: wanting the best for someone, and taking the necessary steps to carry that out. The *New Law* is about caring for everyone including God because we are all One. This means no matter who they are, we do our best to take the best action for everyone. This is what it would mean to let the selfishness of human behavior go. It is selfishness which destroys all of us. That is all global warming is about. Global Warming is nothing but the desire for energy and the money produced by that energy, and this selfishness could kill us all, but the only way for everyone to have virtue in any society would be to have everyone in that society practice love and selflessness. All could agree that love is the universal moral; so, it should not be the pseudo-morals that so many of us live by.

It is also the pseudo-laws of a societies which are meant to control the hand as stated above, but people in societies need their hands controlled in order for people to live with each other because a lot of people will not take the right actions because all life suffers from this selfishness and very few of us even look at our own minds. This is the problem of the human psyche, and in fact the psyche of all life, but it is the humans that are the "rational" ones on this planet, so we have the biggest problem. Most humans are well known not to live by the *New Law*, even if they claim they do, and very few in history have been able to live by the *New Law* perfectly; therefore, every one of the flesh has their sins.

I would say it is my desire to practice the *New Law* that has been able to get me to be at peace with myself and everything which happened in my life at a young age. I have come to see what happened to me as a child happened. It is over. I explained it in the poems I opened the book with, such as *That Might Be Me i Hate*. I wrote those poems locked up as a child because of all the hatred I had for one man in particular. Because of him, I took that hate out on everyone around me. Not just the man I wanted to kill, but everyone. That man I wanted to kill was my father. The desire I would argue was just a cry for help that I did not understand at anyway at the time, and I was angry at my mother for keeping me in the middle of it.

I was an extremely angry child. I do not think I would have killed anyone because I reach out to a teacher to show him a letter I wrote. It was about being judged and abused as a kid. Both my parents judged me for my disabilities, and I hated my mother for sending me to that detentionary boarding school in the middle of Provo Utah. Today I see she had no option because I was so out of control. She did the best she could just like my father did, as in the Socratic quote above: "nobody would knowing do wrong," but that school, Discovery Academy, screwed my life up even more than it was already. It was at Discovery Academy that I began to truly hate everyone!

Today I do not blame either of my parents for anything and am grateful my mother taught me how to love so well as a young child. She truly cared more than anyone. More so than most mother's I would say. I see today we all just have the same two problems: ignorance and understanding, and if you are the only person with the power of "choice" in your life there is nobody to resent. If there is nobody to resent, you are not a miserable person. This Maya is just our perfect teacher. I have come to believe in the power of metaphysics and can see such things as the *Law of Karma* and the *Theory of Evolution* both tell the same thing: the only thing that remains constant is change and we all either learn or we suffer. If we are happy and filled with love for everything just needing teach us something we can always be happy, but I was someone who could not see this and did not talk to my father for about 18 years after I got sent to my first psych-ward.

When I did decide to get in contact with my father, I had moved up to Portland to live with my mother for a little bit. I was sober for about 4 years at the time and had let go of a lot of my anger. People in recovery showed me what the solution was. That solution was love and forgiveness, and in my first book, *A Vicious Cycle*, I end with the prayer of Saint Francis, which I truly believe gives me the right action for every situation of my life if I want true happiness: "by self-forgetting one finds" and "to love is to be loved." It was the people in recovery that showed me what I needed, and what I needed was their solution of love, forgiveness, and self-improvement.

Some people in recovery are so hell bent on the fact that the *Big Book* is not the *Bible*, but the one thing I realized is the *Big Book* came from the *Bible*. Bill W. based all his arguments on the Oxford Group. The Oxford Group based everything on the *Bible*, and in the 1930s in

America I would not think there would be any other spiritual books of reference that were that handy anyways. There's nothing wrong with a text which preaches love to everyone. I enjoy reading parts of the *Bible* today. I am a Hindu today, and one of the premises of Hinduism is all religions have "truths" to them. I find parts of Hinduism I disagree with too like any form of caste system or being a vegetarian. We need to eat meat and other animal products for our health, and I am against all forms of human racial discrimination as well. I do also agree with the respect for Mother Nature though and there needs to be rights for animals as well, but it is in the *Book of Matthew* which made me realize the only *Law* there truly is, is the *Law of Love*.

In *The Sermon On The Mount* Jesus states:

[17]*"Do not think that I have come to abolish the Law or the Prophets; I have not come to abolish them but to fulfill them.* [18] *For truly I tell you, until heaven and earth disappear, not the smallest letter, not the least stroke of a pen, will by any means disappear from the Law until everything is accomplished.* [19]*Therefore anyone who sets aside one of the least of these commands and teaches others accordingly will be called least in the kingdom of heaven, but whoever practices and teaches these commands will be called great in the kingdom of heaven.* [20]*For I tell you that unless your righteousness surpasses that of the Pharisees and the teachers of the law, you will certainly not enter the kingdom of heaven."*.

The Pharisees were the Jewish ruling class. It was these laws of the Pharisees Jesus has come to abolish. These laws in themselves are the pseudo-laws because they were not the laws based on *The Sermon On The Mount*. The laws of the Pharisees were laws which were meant to rule the Jews and keep them in line under the Roman rule. The Pharisees were given this power by the Romans. The Pharisees' laws were RCBA; therefore, pseudo-laws. They benefited the Pharisees because the Pharisees imposed them to benefit the Romans, so the Romans gave the Pharisees special rights and privileges, these privileges even harmed other Jewish people, and that is why the Pharisees crucified

Jesus. The Pharisees crucified Jesus to get rid of him so they could keep their privileges.

Just like the laws of the Pharisees, the pseudo-laws of a society are based on the RCBA. Laws of any society are specific to their constituents. The laws of *Roe vs. Wade*, *Michigan vs. EPA*, and *Matal vs. Tam* are meant to rule the hand. It is this negation of what solves every problem, and that which is the cure to one's difficulties, that shows pseudo-laws are meant for people in a society. But the pseudo-laws will not lead "all" to happiness and will not lead to the "Kingdom of Heaven." Heaven, for me, is here on earth when the *New Law* is practiced. It is in the moment because Consciousness is all there truly is, and it is the Law of the *New Testament* that shows anyone what they need to do to get to Heaven and be happy here on earth, and that is: "Love thy God, thy Neighbor, and thy Enemy as thyself." It is this law which is the only true law, and this law is the law has led to my happiness.

I have found my peace in finally being able to love my enemy. That man I wanted to kill, as I stated, was my father, and my father was my enemy was my greatest enemy by far for a large part of my life. Hating him made it so I hated myself most of all, and I took that anger out on the world as a child. I fought the whole world because of him. That man taught me two things extremely well when I was a child: I was worthless and how to feel superior to anyone. Those two character defects were perfected at Discovery Academy, and Discovery Academy was what perfected those character defects in my adult life.

When I moved up to Portland back in 2009, I got curious to see my father, just to meet him and get to know him. I had let all of that anger go because of love I had gotten from other people who suffered from their addictions. I had no expectations of what he would be like. I admitted I truly would not know until it happened.

I met him at a restaurant. I still recognized him. When I got the restaurant, he was waiting for me at the bar. He had a beer in his hand. It did not bother me because it does not bother me if anyone drinks or does drugs. Their drinking and drug use is about them, not me, and

I can be around drinking and drug use with no problem because my sobriety is not contingent on anything except my God. If I rely on God, I should not have a problem facing anything. If I rely on God, I do not need to have any anger or any problems because the *Law of Love* is the key to happiness in any circumstance.

He was there drinking, I met him, and we talked. We had a great dinner because of the conversation and food. I just got to let him know a little bit about myself, and since I set any expectations or judgments aside, I enjoyed getting to know him.

After that dinner I would see him quite often when I was living in Portland, and when I moved back down to San Francisco I would call him all the time. He showed a genuine interest in me. He wanted to know what I was doing with my life and what it was that made me happy. I impressed him with my education, and he thought it was great what I was doing. He had no expectations or judgments about me at all. He even told me how intelligent I was all the time. He said once to me "you seem to be smarter than I am." That man would never say that to anyone unless he meant it too.

He was about 65 when I got to know him. He did drugs, drank, and smoked for about 50 years, so he was not long for this planet. I moved back to San Francisco to marry my wife after about nine months in Portland, and it was about 10 years of staying in touch with him before he died.

When he got sick, it was at that time in my life I started to tell him I loved him over the phone every time I talked with him, and I would call him every day. He would even tell me he loved me. "I love you" were three words that took most of my life to say to anyone after my childhood, but I went up to Portland during spring break to see him one last time and tell him to his face I loved him. I even had no problem hugging him.

When I got to recovery, I could not even give anyone a hug. People would try and give me a hug, and I would be extremely mean and cruel to them. After coming to recovery for 15 years I eventually started to be able to give people hugs. After going to recovery for 15 years I could say I love you to a select amount of people, then, after a little while, I could say it to anyone. I could not say I love you to anyone without me needing to hear it back, or without the fear that I might not hear it back. I was always so scared of people rejecting me, and that is why I could not say it to people even if I felt it. If I told someone I loved them, and I did not hear it back, I felt so worthless that it terrified completely, so I could not say it to anyone at all for a large portion of my life and it was very painful.

People in my family do not say "I love you" to each other too often. I have noticed with myself love was the only thing I ever wanted from anyone. I believe love is all any of us truly want from the people in our lives. Admitting that all we want is love just also scares lots of people because it exposes us and makes us all vulnerable. It is the fear of getting hurt which kept me from giving what I wanted away, and like Jesus taught, love is the only thing which will cure us all. Love is the bases for the only the only true law, and laws of a society are meant for controlling the hand; so, if someone lives by the only law there truly is: The *Law of Love*, then the hand is controlled quite easily by the mind. The pseudo-laws of a society are not needed only if the mind is controlled, but the *Law of Love* is an extremely difficult law to practice perfectly. To perfect the *Law of Love* would be for all of us to understand all our thoughts at every single moment. I would argue the reason most do not do it too well because most of us are not even paying attention to what we are truly thinking. Yet doing the right thing does not need to be a struggle when the *Law of Love* is understood and practiced like Socrates stated virtues need to be in the actions we take. When we do this, the conflicts in life disappear.

I am no longer a miserable suicidal person. I no longer live in his shadow or am plagued with the torture and the shackles of my mind. I am free and happy all because I can love anyone today, even my father without resentment. Loving others freely allows me to love myself. I do not need to be scared of anyone when I live by this. I also hardly see doctors anymore and I do not even have a psychiatrist. I have been on almost every psychiatric medication in the PDR at one time.

I live my life quite freely today. I no longer need to ruin my life and the lives of others around me because I feel like I will never get love or be accepted. To be free of fear and hate is an amazing experience. Especially when it has controlled you and destroyed everything in your life at one time. I can be happy no matter what, today, all because of the *Law of Love*.

The best way I have found to look at human motivation is through the book *I Am That, Talks with Sri Nisargadatta Maharaj*. He opened my eyes to the only true motivation we all have, and how to forgive anyone: "Life is love and love is life. What keeps the body together but love? What is desire but the love of self? What is fear but the urge to protect? What is knowledge but the love of truth? The means and form may be wrong, but the motive behind is always love - love of the me and the mine. The me and the mine may be small and insignificant, or may explode and embrace the universe, but love remains" (Nisargadatta P68). It was this quote that enabled me to see what everyone's motivations are at their core is love; even my father's when I was a child. As a child my father had a desire for alcohol, and as Nisargadatta points out, all desire is nothing but a love of self. That love of alcohol was nothing but a misguided form of the love, and is a selfish desire, and all pseudo-morals and pseudo-laws are just misguided forms of the True Law: the *Law of Love*. They are based on a love of self, or a love of the few. Instead of the Love of All. If you want to forgive someone just realize that their motive behind all actions is nothing but love in the wrong form, that wrong form of love is a misunderstanding and in ignorance, just like Socrates said.

I met a girl in a meeting who sexually abused her younger half-brother. That girl sexual abused him because she was raped by her mother's boyfriend. She told me that she left the house because her stepmother kept strangling her unconscious over and over because her stepmother found out, and she broke the rules of her stepmother's house. She was a kid at the time and only did to the brother what was done to her. That is nothing but the *Law of Karma*, which is nothing but the *Law of Cause and Effect*, or Newton's *Law of Reciprocity*. There are amazing articles I have read that show anyone that the *Law of Love* and the *Law of Karma* are basically the same thing. The only difference is the *Law of Karma* does not judge. With the *Law of Karma*, I take an action, these are my consequences. Every action just has a result, which is nothing but reciprocity, but both the *Law of Karma* and the *Law of Love* tell us that if we act out of anger more, anger will be created. If someone acts out of love, more love will be created, and the only way to fight anger is with love. This was the same message as Thoreau, Gandhi, and Dr. King, which they all based on the *Book of Matthew*.

When you realize love is everyone's constant motivation, be it a misguided or misunderstood form of love, you can forgive anyone. It is amazing what awareness will do for anyone. Awareness is 99.9% of the problem for all of us, and is why I meditate daily for 45 minutes as shown in my chapter on ADHD. The reason that girl got strangled unconscious by her stepmother, is her stepmother had a love for her son, and wanted to be able to control and protect the other child. The stepmother loved her son and didn't want to lose her son to the state, yet the stepmother lost all control because her fear did not let her understand the situation in anyway. This is what Nisargadatta meant when he stated above: "what is fear but the urge to protect?" Fear is a natural emotion we all misuse.

This is the same thing that is happening in the Middle East. There are those who love Israel and those who love Palestine. One has a fear they will lose something; one has a fear that they will not get it back: the Holy Land. Not getting something one desires, or losing something someone has, are the two types of fears; how those two types of fear manifest is anger: "The means and the form may be wrong, but the motive behind is always love" as Nisargadatta stated above.

I have had a couple of people say I have saved their lives, and I'm the reason they believe in God. It was not that difficult. Anyone can do it. There is this one lady who has had a lot of brain damage from strokes. I did not really know her too well before the strokes at all, but one day I saw her suffering. She was in a wheelchair saying she just wanted to die. I went up and said hi to her. It was at that moment I started to spend time with her. Not a lot of time, but I just made an effort to see her once a week for a while. All I do today is talk to her and say hi on the phone. I text her and tell her I love her throughout the week. It is so simple. Anyone can do it. I have found it is the only thing any of us truly want. Anyone can make a difference in someone else's life: Anyone! And it feels wonderful to make a positive difference in someone's life.

It was the Saints, like Augustine and Pseudo-Dionysius, which got me back to Catholicism. I wrote how I am a basically a Neoplatonist too. Hinduism and Neoplatonism have lots and lots in common as well, and Neoplatonism is what all the Catholic Saints were in the Middle Ages too. It was these Saints which got me to see the only law, which is truly a law, is the same law that works for everyone: the *Law of Love*, which is nothing but a judgement on the *Law of Karma*: the only thing which remains constant is change and we either learn or we suffer.

When my father was dying, I got to hug him and tell him I loved him over and over. I have said it to my sisters and all my family members, and sometimes they do not even say it back to me. They do not need to. It is fine. I have no need for the fear of rejection, so I just let it all go. Today I try and live by the only true moral there is: love. This only true moral is what makes the only true law there is. With this law there is no RCBA's because there are no winners and losers. Anyone who practices this law will win, and every life that person touches wins as well because when the mind is controlled the hand will follow. Other lives are not damaged by another people's hands when the *Law of Love* is practiced.

Jesus showed love for the Pharisees who were nailing him to the cross. If I am going to be happy, then just like Jesus, it does not matter what anyone else does. It only matters what I do, and no matter what they do, the only thing I should try and do is love them. I am not a Saint, and I still have a long way to go. I mess up all the time at this, but through awareness, and daily practice, I am able to change my habits. Most of what we all do is nothing but habitual, as I prove through the rest of this book, so I still have a hard time loving everyone in all circumstances. I will tell anyone though it has gotten easier the more I have practiced it. The rest of this book is about developing new thinking and behaviors to overcome one's mental illness; so, the *Law of Love* will work for anyone, be you a Christian or not because all religions have "truths" to them.

I also point out to Christians in America all the time that I do not see how the *2nd Amendment* and the *Law of Love* are compatible. They seem shocked and confused. It seems quite obvious and simple to me. But none of them want to even see it. I have terrified just pointing out this simple truth to them, and as I stated most of what we do is just habit and awareness is 99.9% of the problem. The greatest person to practice the *Law of Love* of the 20th century was not even a Christian. It was Gandhi. Gandhi studied Thoreau, and Thoreau himself was pro-Christ and anti-Christian, because the Christians themselves have never practiced the principles of Christ all that well. Gandhi said it best, "I like your Christ. I do not like your Christians. Your Christians are not much like your Christ." Modern Christians are still trying to reconcile the *Old Law* and the *New Law*, which leads to nothing but insanity in an empirical world where people deny paradoxes. Most humans also have no desire to look at their own mind or their own actions, which is what pride keeps us all from doing, and pride is their greatest sin as well.

If one looks at modern non-violent peaceful protest in America it is based on Dr. Martin Luther King Jr. Dr. King based it on Gandhi; So, when one thinks about it, even gay rights are based on the spirit of Christ. They are based on the abolitionist interpretation of the *Book of Matthew*: All non-violent peaceful protest is about showing love for your enemy because anger only breads more anger. This is all nothing but a radical interpretation of the *Book of Matthew*, and it is nothing but a simple logical conclusion, which most of us refuse to acknowledge.

The most articulate of the 2020 Presidential candidates, Mayor Pete Buttigeig has stated, "Christians in this country hide behind the clock of religion. They claim to praise the principles of loving your God and your enemy just as themselves, but they don't live by it." Karl Marx said the same thing about the colonialist. Lots of people get pride and humility confused, and that is because they get fear and faith confused. The reason for this is that people want the impossible: certainty in an uncertain world. That would be the only reason one would try to reconcile the *Old* and *New Laws*, and the only reason anyone takes a literal interpretation of their scriptures. These people are not after what is true, but they are after holding what they have believed their whole lives to be true, which is nothing but pride.

If someone wants what is true, they need to always admit when they are wrong, and we are all wrong constantly about the conclusions we come to in this empirical world (Maya). People always want the impossible. The reason we are all wrong all the time is because the only constant state is a state of change; therefore, uncertainty in this empirical world. If we want what is certain that it is only uncertainty or the God of the *Rgveda*, because that God is only defined consciousnesses, and every experience I have proves to me one thing constantly: that I am a conscious Being. Just like every experience we all have proves to all of us we are conscious beings. What those experiences truly are, are all up for debate. Those experiences only validate one thing: existence! Everything else in this empirical world I dedicated my mind to try and understand, and the one thing it has shown to me over and over is that I need to constantly admit all of my errors because we all have lot of them. It is only through acknowledging our error that we learn, which is what the *Law of Karma* is all about: learning, and I either learn or I suffer by the actions I take, and as Gandhi stated: "if everyone did an eye for an eye, the whole world would be blind." That is exactly why the *2nd Amendment* and the *Law of Love* are not compatible. The anger and hatred needs to end with me in my life and you in your life.

There was a movie that was released in 2017 that got best picture that made this same argument. Everyone I talked to seem to think it was some new retackle argument. The movie was *Three Billboards*.

In this movie this mother loses her child to a murderer. She blames the town sharif for her anger and that murder just of her child just creates more and more anger. It is the oldest of all arguments and it even shown in ancient scriptures that originated in different continents. Anger just creates more anger. Just as the daughter getting strangled by her stepmother did, which only happened because the girl got sexually abused herself. Just learn to understand and forgive.

Today I take all religions as having "truths." Some speak the "truth" more than others, but most are not practiced very well. Most of the followers of every religion get things like fear and faith confused. There is a lack of understanding about their principles because most people do not want to put forth the effort to truly understand their religion, and to truly practice their religion.

According to Pope Francis, the Kingdom of Heaven is open to anyone no matter their God or their religion. All you have to do is have a rational mind and love your neighbor and your enemy as yourself, and if we truly want that then, when the mind is controlled, then the hand will follow. When someone does that, then happiness will follow because God is everything and we are all One. This also means the root of everything, in every action we all take, is nothing but love. As Nisargadatta Maharaj says, "Wisdom tells me I am Nothing. Love tells me I am everything. In between the two my life flows."

CHAPTER 4

The Power of Inaction

THE REST OF THIS BOOK is going to be about combining ancient philosophy and modern science. I will be using the medical theory of the neuroplasticity of the human brain and fuse it together with the mental exercises of *Ancient Vedic* scriptures. Neuroplasticity is why I was able to finally learn how to read at the age of thirty that I wrote about in the chapter *A Glimmer of Hope*. Reading was something which seemed like I was completely incapable of doing for most of my life because of my learning disabilities. The neuroplasticity of the human brains is saying this empirical world is constantly changing and shifting and all our minds (brains) should be built to continually develop throughout our lives in a positive way which helps us adapt to those shifts and changes that are constantly appearing in front of all of us. My thesis that I proved in the last chapter *Pseudo-Laws and Pseudo-Morals*: when the mind is controlled, the hand will follow, is what jnana yoga is all about. Jnana in Sanskrit means knowledge or mind. What yoga means in Sanskrit is practice, so in the rest of this book I show how I am able to understand mine. By me understanding my mind, and the tricks I have taught myself using ancient principles, which apply to us all, I infer others can use these same tools in this book to help themselves with their mental illnesses and brain function difficulties because I have had a lot of brain dysfunctions I have overcome besides just learning how to read. When I combined modern theories with ancient philosophy of the mind it has led me to true happiness. True happiness is what I want for everyone these days.

In this chapter I have my theory of the minds which is where I prove that I am not really that much different than anyone else using ancient philosophy and the psychology of modern movies and commercials. Sure, I have a rare organic brain disorder, which gives me the aspects of eight different disorders without fitting one stereotype, but ancient scriptures and religions are meant for everyone, so are catchy commercials and entertaining movies. I have learned how to understand my mind and get off most of my medications through combining all kinds of principles which are meant for everyone. My hope is that others can use these same tools to help themselves understand their own minds with their mental health issues. I am also not encouraging anyone to get off medication. It took me years of doing these exercises daily and I have to continue to do them. I argue in favor of modern science throughout this whole book. My hope is that everyone can better understand their own minds and improve their realities no matter what their reality is because, as I state all throughout this book: our realities are nothing but what we perceive, and our minds are nothing but imagination. As I also prove in my chapter on overcoming schizophrenia: we all have false beliefs, and it is the really crazy people that have no ability to question their sanity, so "insanity" applies to most of us because most people I have noticed have no ability to question their own sanity! We all struggle with pride, which is the greatest of all sins for the very reason it tells us we are right when the only thing anyone can be truly certain of is their own existence! "I am" is the main premises of *Vedic Philosophy*.

I take medication still to this day. I am on CBD for my epilepsy, which I would argue has some mild psychoactive effects for attention deficit issues. If I need to take other psychiatric medications again for psychosis or anything else, I will. I just show in this book how I have been able to get off all my psych medications through understanding my own mind in a daily practice of single pointed concentration med-itation (Trataka). Yet, my true hope is that I can get anyone reading this to reflect and look for similarities if they feel as though they are mentally ill or not. I also encourage anyone to better understand their own mind in the combined processes of jnana yoga and modern science if they struggle with mental health or not. I am a firm believer that everyone can help their minds and their realities through a daily practice Trataka outlined in my chapter on ADHD.

I would not say we are all identical in the empirical aspects, but I would argue we all have much more in common with each other than anyone of us might first think. Even someone with my organic brain disorder, which is quite a rare condition: hetero-topic grey matter. As I want to reiterate, I am not a doctor, nor do I argue anyone should not be on medication. I am all for Western Science, which is what got me into Hinduism to being with. I have found all the different forms Hinduism, especially Vedanta, are extremely compatible with modern science, and as of today, nothing has helped my mental state more than the practice that I developed through *Ancient Vedic* scriptures. These are all reinforced in the book *I Am That*. Nisargadatta Maharaj, who the book *I Am That* is about his transcribed conversations with people who sought his council, is my modern day Masai if I have one.

I have also been on almost every psych-medication and anticonvulsant in the PDR up till the year I got off of SSDI, which was something like 2017 I believe? I was on SSDI for over ten years myself, and today, the only medication I am taking is the CBD for my epilepsy. Every once in a while, I take 1/8 of a 5mg tablet of Saphris, which is an anti-psychotic medication, just to sleep, but it is only for sleep. I don't take enough for Saphris to be in my system for the full 24 hours. The minimum dose is 5mg taken twice daily, and I cut one 5mg tablet into eight pieces just to sleep for 6 hours or so. Sleeping is something I have struggled with my whole life because parts of my brain naturally over produce dopamine, which is what happens to schizophrenics and bipolars, which one of my diagnoses schizoaffective-bipolar type. Schizoaffective is a combination of both schizophrenia and bipolar, but they are considered higher functioning than a paranoid schizophrenic.

What got me off all those psychiatric medications is the way I meditate daily. Specifically, this meditation is outlined in Chapter 6 of the *Bhagavad-Gita* and reiterated in lots of *Vedic* scriptures, such as the *Mandukya Upanishad*. I haven't had a psych-medication prescription fill in years. I hardly take any medication today and I can think clearly, work full time, write, give presentations, and participate well in society. These were things I was completely incapable of doing for years in my life even while taking lot so medications.

Despite the rare congenital defects in my brain: heterotopic grey matter, I do believe others can improve their lives too even if they want to stay on, or need to be on, their medications for the rest of their lives using these mental exercises. Meditation is also good for every human brain, and all our realities, as I will prove throughout this book. I would argue there are two disorders that I delt with that I am sure others can completely overcome without medication with the way I meditate: ADHD and panic attacks.

Remember, no human is born with an "IQ," for lack of a better term, being that "IQ" educational, emotional, or social. Developing our minds all throughout our lives is what neuroplasticity is all about. Our brains (minds) are meant to continually adapt throughout our lives, which is why I am sure that people can overcome their ADHD without such terrible drugs as Ritalin. I have talked to doctors who specialize in childhood psychology who think that Ritalin is the worst drug that is prescribed in anyway with all the damage it does to the brain. With such diagnoses as ADHD, which is more developmental, anyone who can get off such toxic drugs as Ritalin should get off them. Ritalin, and the different forms of Ritalin, are nothing but speed. Speed, by far, causes more damage to the brain than any other drug which can be abused. Ritalin can cause issues even just through proper use just like all other medications can. Ritalin seems to be nothing but a poison to me.

Benzodiazepines are drugs that are most commonly used for anxiety and are by far one of the most addictive drugs for any addict. The withdrawals for Benzodiazepines can be fatal. Sure, they use them in emergency situations to stop seizures and things like panic attacks, but I have seen people die from seizures because of their withdrawals from different benzodiazepines. No type of Benzodiazepines ever really even worked for me more than once no matter how much I took, which shows my abnormalities and tolerances to all kinds of drugs, but the theory in this book can help anyone improve their lives because the biggest problem with all humanity is ignorance and understanding as I proved in *Pseudo-Laws and Pseudo-Morals*. Ignorance and understanding are out biggest issues because love is the root cause of every action we all take. We just get confused with what we are truly supposed to be doing in the moment. We just do not see the root of fear is love: fear we will lose something we love or fail to get a desire met. If we want to be able to take the first step in anything, we have to see what the problem is, so we need awareness. If anyone wants more awareness, the true key is an ancient solution: daily meditation. Especially the thinning of the mind and being able to drop it completely like I show in my chapter on ADHD through single pointed concentration meditation (Trataka).

Lots of the answers to the human mind, and my key to happiness, are in these ancient scriptures of the *Vedas* because all humans, in fact all life, have the same basic desire and are driven by the same forces: pleasure and pain. We are all controlled by the desires of what we love. Love is just the root of every desire and the pleasures we seek. These desires and pleasures are nothing but the love of ourselves. Just realize, 99.9% of all human DNA is identical, so no matter how different we take ourselves to be, we all have a lot more in common with each other than lots of us like to acknowledge. In fact, all life shares a lot of the same DNA because humans share over 100 genomes of other forms of life. I truly have found myself to have a lot more in common with anyone and everything than I ever thought possible once I opened my mind.

Our "IQ's," (intelligence) is based on two things beyond our control: genetics and circumstances; 90% of what someone learns happens in the first five years of their life. Given the right information and motivation, we can do lots for ourselves to get our brains to continue to develop and grow throughout our lives. I have even been able to overcome mild brain damage from my seizures and drug abuse through exercising my mind every day as well.

16 years ago, when I got sober, I could not really remember too much because of the seizure I had from speed abuse and my epilepsy combined. Today I am a savant again with my memory. I can demonstrate my memory to anyone if they like, and it was all through my mental exercises and the Neurological Evaluation I had done at UCSF. I have also met others who have had brain damage and brain surgeries, where pieces of their brains were removed, and doctors said they were not going to ever have that high of a level of intelligence, but I have seen two of these other people defy their doctors and get such things as college degrees and graduate at the top of their class.

ॐ

In the Ancient Indian philosophy of Vedanta, it is the Gunas which make up everything. In the micro sense, the three Gunas are what make up the different pieces of the mind. The three Gunas are Rajas, Tames, and Sattva. Rajas has to do with things like passion, anger, and all kinds of misguided energy. Tamas has to do with things like depression, delusions, and darkness. The Rajas itself has its roots in the Tamas because of the states of delusion, and the misinterpretation of what truly is. Then there is Sattva. The Sattva is the ground of Being that is in God. The Sattva is within us all, and the Sattva is the ideal goal we should all get closer too when it comes to our minds.

I am also using identity theory in this book. In identity theory the brain and the mind are the same thing. This is made obvious to us when there is damage to the brain, this impedes our thoughts and actions, and in Vedanta the mind is made of thoughts and is truly nothing but imagination. To get the mind closer to Sattva would be the goal for anyone in this religion, yet for most of my life, because of all of my physical abuse as a child, and enhanced by my psychological disorders, as well as the trauma I got from Discovery Academy, the thoughts of my mind had mostly been cluttered with Rajas and Tamas. I realized if I was going to address the thoughts of my mind and get myself closer to a pure state of Sattva, the best thing to do was to not focus on what is important, or Sattva, but to focus on what is not important the Rajas and Tamas. This means I need to find the thoughts I should let go of, and upon seeing which of my thoughts I should let go of I would detaching from Rajas and Tamas completely. I could then get my mind closer and closer to Pure Sattva and allow the Sattva to control me completely.

Executive function has to do with the part of the brain which is rational, discursive, and which regulates emotions. My brain has been in a constant state of high executive dysfunction for a large part of my life. I have the aspects of eight different mental disorders without fitting one stereotype: epilepsy, schizoaffective bipolar type, obsessive-compulsive personality, ADD, dyslexia, borderline autism, general anxiety and PTSD, and I've struggled with suicidal depression throughout my life starting at a very, very young age. I have no ability to count how many times I ended up in a psych ward for trying to kill myself. A lot of those suicide attempts were for attention and other times I meant it and tried hard. I just never died.

I have been diagnosed with aspects of all these disorders without fitting one stereotype because of my rare heterotopic grey matter that is in my brain. This heterotopic grey matter is the direct cause of my seizures. I had a Neurological Evaluation at UCSF, by Brandon E. Kopald, Psy.D., that states my brain is constantly going in and out of eight different brain states from moment to moment. A brain state is a level of what anyone brain is function at in any given moment. This is abnormal to have someone's brain constantly jumping in and out of different states, let alone eight of them. I would argue most people function in a single brain state for large parts of their lives. My brain, during this test, was jumping in and out from moment to moment. These brain states are not identical to the eight different disorders I have been diagnosed with, but anyone could see how this executive dysfunction of the eight different brain states would directly influence these disorders and make me incapable of treatment for a large part of my life. Most doctors I met had no ability to help me in any way, and lots of doctors made my life worse from a very young age. Especially the doctor I saw at Discovery Academy.

I based this essay on years of psychological hospitalizations and this Neurological Evaluation at UCSF by Dr. Kopald at UCSF, done on 09/14/2017, which is what showed my brain is constantly jumping between these eight different brains states. The brain states that my brain were constantly jumping between, were a majority of the states of Rajas to Tamas in my opinion for a large part of my life. The proof of that is my Oppositional Defiance Disorder I was locked up for as a child. I took that difficult behavioral issue and it was perpetuated throughout a large part of my adult life as well, but it was doctor at UCSF: Dr. Paul Garcia, who is head of epileptology, who diagnosed me with the heterotopic grey matter. A heterotopic grey matter is a nerve which can be seen on an MRI. This nerve is adjacent to my right later ventral and in my right frontal horn of my brain, which causes the seizures and speculated to cause, and definitely influences, these other disorders.

Three of my disorders aren't really about my brain jumping in and out of brain states: dyslexia, ADHD, and autism. The dyslexia, has to do with parts of my brain being underdeveloped, and parts of my brain being over developed, and they have a hard time communicating. This confusion of communication are also characteristics of ADHD and autism.

Autism and ADHD in fact have a lot of the same symptoms. Lots of doctors have speculated recently that ADD and ADHD really are just a mild form of autism. I agree that ADHD is just a mild form of autism. It is also why it is impossible to get an appointment at the autism clinic at UCSF because more and more people are getting diagnosed with it, and nobody, no matter who we are, has a 180 social "IQ" in anyway. Every single person has autistic characteristics. I work daily to ease the symptoms of both the ADHD and autism. This daily effort is also about the development of parts of my brain that are underdeveloped just like interpreting written symbols which is the issue with dyslexia. I will go into that more in the chapter on brain damage and in the next chapter on ADHD.

The autism is an organic disorder which affects my ability to relate to others, but even that is abnormal when it comes to my brain. I am very good with people when they are suffering, but I am terrible with the average individual just socializing. Even my epilepsy is abnormal with the frequency of my seizures and the patterns of their occurrences, as well as the abnormal and atypical reactions to anticonvulsants and other medications I have been on. This is what made it so that I was undiagnosed with epilepsy for five years as a child. My seizures were so abnormal, and I was so difficult to deal with, that the doctors at Discovery Academy told everyone I was doing it for attention. The doctors at Discovery Academy were still quite terrible doctors, and by far the worst I ever saw. That opinion was reinforced when I had talked to other kids from Discovery Academy years after I left, and the medications that doctor had those other kids on were all wrong for them too. Every single one I talked to, and I talked to lots of them, all told me the doctor there was completely terrible and made their life worse.

My seizures are definitely a structural abnormality. This nerve gives a surge of chemicals at the time I am having a seizure. A seizure itself is nothing but a surge of electricity in the brain. This surge of electricity will also fluctuate the chemicals in the brain, because all our brains function off of nothing but electricity, and all any chemical is, is nothing but a compound of electromagnetic energy. Yet, only about 2% of the people with epilepsy have a heterotopic grey matter. It is hard to know how many people suffer from a heterotopic grey matter because some people might have it and it is too small to see on the MRI. I stated that my heterotopic grey matter in my brain is located adjacent to my right lateral ventricle and in my right frontal horn, and with this surge of chemicals happening in my brain from the seizures, it shows at least a part of all of these disorders to be an organic executive brain disfunction, but all mental illnesses are both genetics and circumstances no matter who we are.

Mental illness being a combination of both genetics and circumstances is proven by studying identical twins. Just because one of the twins gets an organic disorder, such as paranoid schizophrenia, it does not mean the other one will. They are both born with the same genes, but as they get older, their genes mutate, so their genes change just like everyone else's over their lives. Their genes mutate differently because of the different circumstances they are in. The identical twins' genomes are not anywhere near identical when they are measured at ages such as 60, so circumstances play a role even in organic brain disorders such as paranoid schizophrenia.

My Seizures were also brought upon by circumstances at Discovery Academy. The kids there would try and pass each other out to get a quick buzz. One time when they cut off my oxygen supply is when I had my first grand mal seizure. It is this lack of oxygen to my brain is what triggered my seizure to begin with at the age of 16 or so, even though I had the nerve in my head my whole life. When I have this surge of chemicals in my brain from the seizures, this surge influences both the brain states and the thoughts. I noticed this because I sit in silent meditation every day for forty-five minutes and just watch my thoughts.

I just happened to start the daily meditation right before I had this Neurological Evaluation. I saw, after I had the Neurological Evaluation at UCSF, that when my brain states were jumping extremely rapidly at the same time my thoughts were bouncing all over the place too. I would also argue that there are times my brain could be jumping in and out of even more or less brain states than the eight brain states this specific Neurological Evaluation showed because of my constant fluctuations with seizure and moods. I even have prolonged cycles of the mania as well, which I was not manic, and on lots of medication, at the time of the Neurological Evaluation at UCSF.

My seizures, as well as such things as mania, come in swings and waves, which is a direct relation to the diagnosis of bipolar. This bipolar is connected directly to my mood. But I noticed in silent meditation that when my thoughts would change rapidly, so would my feelings along with all other such issues such as more seizures within that 24-hour period. I have noticed since I have been digging deeper into my subconscious with meditation, every time I switch to another brain state there is a shift in thinking which goes along with it. It was an extremely rapid change when this all first began. I also enjoy meditation now, which was definitely not how it started out, and it is only this practice of daily meditation, explicitly laid out in the next chapter on ADHD, which has gotten me to let go of Rajas and Tamas that make up these brain states and disorders my brain is mostly made of, improving my life, and becoming more and more Sattvic.

The thoughts of my mind, and anyone's mind (brain), are made from the three Gunas, yet my mind is in a constant change of brain states and executive brain dysfunction. So, do the brains states precede the thoughts, or do the thoughts precede the brain states? Was the first question I asked myself when I sat in silence after I was told the results of this Neurological Evaluation. There are also the feelings which change with the brain states that are triggered by the different thoughts. Is it the brain states or the thoughts that influence my emotions? I have had a very hard time finding medications that work like I stated, and I really hate being on medication because of the side-effects and the expense. I took it as impossible for anyone to address their brain disorders without medication at one time. Noticing how much my mind was jumping with the thoughts I asked myself: can I address my brain states and disorders through my thinking? I started to wonder could I focus on my brain states through the Gunas of my mind? Maybe I could redirect my brain states through redirecting my thinking! I did not know it was possible for me to get me off all my medications, and it is that fact that I got off most medications that has gotten me to rewrite this essay and all the chapters in this book countless times! All because I my brain continues to improve!

I have also noticed through meditation (separate from the brain states), that thoughts rise and fall in my mind without any control. I am constantly aware of what I am thinking these days, and thoughts rise and fall in everyone's mind without their control. I only have confirmed this by talking to others who meditate on a daily basis. I was able to shut a Buddhist monk up right away who was convinced she had free will, so I asked her: "it is how we feel about what we think that controls our actions, so do you have any control over the thoughts that rise in your mind and how they make you feel?"

She was in shock! She was giving a Dharma talk at the San Francisco Zen Center at that moment, and she had no response whatsoever to that challenge! She is also someone who watches her own mind every day too, and had been meditating much, much longer than I had, but she couldn't respond to me because I proved to her none of us have any control over the thoughts that rise in our minds and how they make us feel, so how are we supposed to truly have this free will we all claim to function off of?

How and why random thoughts do rise in our minds is something neurologists and psychiatrists still have not discovered the happenings of yet. Sure, certain situations will provoke certain thoughts, but I am sitting in silence, just like anyone else who meditates, just watching these thought rising randomly at different rates triggered by different brain states, and anyone I have talked to has told me they have no control over their minds, especially when they first begin meditation too. I have seen lots of people refuse to meditate for the very reason they have no control over their minds, and they do not like what they see in their mind when they are meditating. It scares them to see how little control they have over their own minds. Yet, these thoughts control the emotions we all feel, and when the emotions are provoked by the thoughts in our daily lives, they are followed by the actions we take.

The epilepsy, schizo, and the autism are not mood disorders, but they directly influence the brain states as well as influence the feelings.

It is the thoughts which control the feelings as well, so it is that the thoughts and the brain states are contingent on each other. If there are thoughts **(T)**, then the brain states **(B)** change, and if there are brain states **(B)**, then the thoughts change **(T)**; it is the change in the brain states and thoughts that control how I feel, and how we all feel **(F)**, which it is how I feel about what I think that controls my actions **(A)**.

The Buddhist monk agreed that her thoughts lead to how she felt, which controlled her actions. She had no understanding of the brain states I am talking about, but it was the testing of the brain states at UCSF, and adding it to the awareness brought upon by daily meditation which got me to the full equation of human behavior: $(((T{>}B){*}(B{>}T)){>}F){>}A$.

The problem with this equation is if the brain states are what are truly coming first, then I, or anyone else, would have no ability to "control" our actions whatsoever. The only way to solve this dilemma would be to make an assumption of faith, which all science does constantly is make assumptions, then verify those assumptions. So, if I simplify the equation by putting my thoughts before the brain states. In symbolic logic if the conjunction is isolated you can just drop one of the premises. So:

$(T{>}B){*}(B{>}T)$

This can be simplified to:

$(T{>}B)$,

Then it can be added back to the rest of the argument:

$((T{>}B){>}F){>}A$.

This equation shows me the best way to deal with my feelings, which control my actions, is to address my thoughts first. I would need to have the thoughts at least influencing my brain states to try and address my disorders through how I consciously think. Using this theory, I have been basically able to get off all my psychiatric pharmaceuticals! It has been amazing because lots of my issues I have been able to overcome doing this! And most of the medications I have tried did nothing for me anyways accept cause problems and money!

What I have noticed is I do not have influence over the thoughts that rise in my brain, but I do have influence over what I do with each thought once they do if I can be truly aware of what I am thinking. The more I train my brain the easier it gets as well. My theory is that I can rewire my brain states, which give direct influence on the different diagnosis: schizoaffective-bipolar type, ADHD, dyslexia, autism, obsessive-compulsive disorder personality, anxiety and PTSD, and depression, if I can see these thoughts for what they are: imagination. I work on emptying my mind daily to get to my pure state of being that is within all of us: consciousness. Today I can function in this society without such medications that keep me on government assistance. It does not need to be the control of the thoughts rising, but the ability to realize a thought is just a thought, or nothing but that imagination, and take these thoughts as something I should take as important or not when I am walking down the street.

One of the most amazing things that I have learned about the mind by sitting in silence is the only thing the mind truly is, is imagination. When someone realizes thoughts are not reality, this realization can take the power right out of any thought. I have been able to do function through mild hypnotic illusion that I still deal with at times. In my past, I have been completely powerless over my actions for most of my life because I have been completely powerless over my thoughts and how these thoughts made me feel. I took this "imagination" as reality. I was powerless over all my thinking because I was never aware of what I was thinking, and my behavior was extremely out of control for a large part of my life.

I don't believe most people have any idea of what they are thinking most of the time because it was Sigmund Fraud that said 90% of the human mind is subconscious, and it was Descartes that said if you meditate you can look at your mind from any angle. Both those concepts are in the *Vedas*, and the *Vedas* have been my answer to things most doctors could not help me with.

ॐ

I have always gotten into a lot of conflict with people throughout my life, and, at times, daily. This was a chronic issue I have had to deal with for most of my life. I was institutionalized as a child for my behavior at Discovery Academy. I brought these behavioral issues into my adult life as well. As a child I had the most extreme case of Oppositional Defiance Disorder I have ever really heard of. It was all verbal, but I had no ability to think something and not say it. It got me into extreme amounts of trouble, but meditation, and developing my brain, extremely slowly, on a daily basis, has been, by far, been the best way to treatment I have ever gotten.

I have been attacked and beaten up more times than I can possibly count for the things that I have said to people. I am someone who has had a doctor in charge of hospital cussed me out for what I have said to them, and I was his patient at the time it happened. A psychiatrist, Richard Shapiro, told me my verbal "IQ" with insults was at a genius level, somewhere around 150 to 160. I have always been able to see what is wrong with anyone, then take their own words that they said to me and use both those against them. I am also quite terrible at seeing what is appropriate and what is not, but nothing makes people angrier than when you get all of their friends to laugh at them. Sometimes I thought I was just joking around, but others took it extremely offensively. Then they would get angry, and I would really go off on them because I would get defensive, but I have been beaten up by people and ended up in the hospital for no other reason than what I have said to them. This has happened more times in my life that I can possibly count. I have even gotten false charges from police officers from what I have said to them. As a child I had the head of the female students in the front office in tears at Discovery Academy screaming "I am not fat!," and Dr. Throne, who owned the place, was cussing at me too! And they were all Mormon! So that F-word was not even allowed for him to say to me, but Dr. Thorne did!

Even when people were pounding my head in, I still could not shut my mouth! One of the other things the Neurological Examination showed me at UCSF is I have never had any impulse control whatsoever, and these thoughts and behaviors of aggression are what make up the Rajas of my mind. Because of the Rajas, and the complete lack of any impulse control, which is an underdevelopment of my brain from the ADHD and autism, if I thought something, I had to say it! Especially if it was rude and funny because I craved the attention so much!

I was completely powerless over what I was thinking and had no impulse control to keep my mouth shut! These thoughts were an exhilaration of nothing but my ego, which in Vedanta is not what I truly am. My biggest addiction by far has been the need to feel superior to another person. That was what was shown by poem I wrote locked up as a kid *That Might Be Me i Hate* in the front of this book. This overpowering ego to be a bully was the extreme pride within me. I was never violent with anyone, but I was an intellectual bully for a large part of my life. All it was, was the fact I was just a very damaged person who was extremely scared of everyone and had no ability to see that fear in anyway. How this fearful character defect manifested was in pride. I loved making everyone feel as stupid and as worthless as my father made me feel.

My father taught me one thing extremely well because, as I wrote above, 90% of what we learn happens in the first five years of our lives. What my father taught me was how to bully anyone. He was both an intellectual and physical bully with me. I was never big enough to beat up anyone at Discovery Academy, but it was at the boarding school I definitely turned into intellectual bully with everyone, which he was to me as well. My father would beat me in chess in three moves when I was in the first grade whenever I tried to play him, and I when I got locked up with those kids at Discovery Academy, I learned how to beat anyone in chess in three moves with my words to keep myself safe. That school made me much worse than just my early childhood alone.

I was getting on the bus a week before I came up with this theory, and there was this African American man who got on the bus with me. His cigarette was still lit so I snapped at him because I hate the smell of cigarette smoke now that I have quit. He looked me up and down, and he got in my face and said something to me. It felt like he was talking down to me. So, while I was pointing my finger directly in his face, I yelled something extremely mean and cruel.

He looked shocked! He was about to get in my face, but then this other African American man started to laugh and said, "Good one!"

Because the other Black guy thought it was so funny, he threw the guy's bag off of the bus to protect me. Because he threw his bag off of the bus, the guy jumped off to go after it. The bus took off and I was safe! This whole interaction would be a state of Rajas in itself.

While this situation was happening, I was extremely scared. I was extremely scared because I am not physically tough as I stated. The consequences of being beaten up have always been overpowered by my ego, pride, zero impulse control, and the value of someone thinking that they are better than me in anyway. These thoughts are nothing except things I take as important, and most of what I took as extremely important was completely self-centered. I have never been able to let my need of superiority go until the last couple of years of me developing this theory, and I am still struggling with it at times, but nothing like I used too. I would argue that the reason I have never been able to let my need go of feeling superior to another person, is because my brain tells me it is so important. Why do I have to take these situations as so important? They do not serve me in any way. They have caused me, and others, harm my whole life. I went off on someone a couple of years ago, and I was terrified the whole time while I was laughing in his face, and that time I ended up in the hospital! But it was drilled into my head in the first five years of my life how to conquer anyone!

After that exact situation, I thought of what I said to the African American on the bus, and I started to laugh really hard. It lifted my mood right up. I started to feel euphoric. I was laughing so hard. Then I started to think about how he treated me, and I started to get really, really angry. I was in a rage. My mood changed in a split second. Then I started to think of my wife and my friends who do not like it when I say those things to people. My wife gets really upset, and when I thought of what her reaction would be I got very sad.

All of these thoughts seem to start a cycle of one brain state to another. They fluctuate so quickly, and it is the same tape that plays on a loop continuing to alter my moods and actions. These same thoughts are constantly being recycled in my head days later; these thoughts do the same thing to my moods every time. I never noticed this my whole life until recently. This is why I completely agree with Freud, that for most of us who do not meditate, 90% of the mind is subconscious, but if anyone wants to see all their thoughts from any angle and what it is that is truly controlling them, I encourage them to sit in silence every single day and meditate, especially Trataka.

With the awareness of my thoughts, and the awareness of the Neurological Evaluation, I have noticed my brain going in very rapid cycles, going from Rajas to Tamas constantly. It was nothing but insanity! An egotistical insanity I had never been able to control because I was never paying attention to any of it!

ॐ

When I was having the Psychological Examination, the lady giving me the test said, "Tell me of as many male names you can think of as possible?"

I responded, "Steven….." then my mind went blank. I felt a little overwhelmed that I could not think of something as simple as male names. I was starting to feel really stupid and was worried about that, so I immediately improvised and said, "Proclus, Plotinus, Theaetetus, Antenor, Pherekydes, Plato, Aristotle, Homer, Virgil, Dante," and I went on like that until she told me to stop. She even complained to me that she did not think she spelled most of the names right with a grunt.

I thought I was so clever, and to this day every time I think of that I start laughing pretty hard. I was told, from the Neurological Examination from UCSF, that my mind is constantly jumping from brain state to brain state, and that is why I paused at first with such an easy question. She also said my "IQ" would be impossible to test because I have so many brain states that my mind is constantly jumping between with this executive dysfunction, but when I think of this specific situation it picks me up and I start to feel euphoric again that I was able to be so clever.

The cleverness is only something I value about myself and then boom: the energy of Rajas! My thoughts and values change, so do my mood. It brings about a hypomania, and I feel completely powerless over it all. I also do not want to control the hypomania when I have it. This hypomania is a surge of the Rajas. I want the hypomania to continue because it feels so good. It is a drug without having to take any chemicals. The same thing that happens to a speed addict and a cocaine addict is what happens to someone who is bipolar and schizophrenic. The chemicals in their brain go up. With me it is especially dopamine that increases just like speed and cocaine. I know this because the medications that have been most effective to stabilize my mood are the dopamine blockers like Saphris, Zyprexa, and Clozaril. All those medications work by keeping anyone's brain from pumping out too much dopamine, and they severally retard thoughts, so it lowers the "IQ." My mind is constantly overactive because of the chemicals are at a higher level.

I was at college, where I was studying philosophy at SFSU, one time just ordering a sandwich and glass of water at a counter not too long ago. I was buying food, and I asked the guy behind the counter, "Could I have a glass of water too? I'll pay for it. I just want a glass."

He was telling me they do not sell glasses of water. I'd have to buy a bottle. So, I said, "They do it everywhere else on campus. I will pay you extra. I just want a glass."

A lady from behind me said, "Don't be a jerk. He said no."

I did not think I was being offensive in any way, but when she said that I went off on her! Other people tried to get in to defend her! I went off on all of them! None of them could keep up with me! I shut them all up, and I was telling them if they wanted this to end all they needed to do was shut up! One lady even took my picture to see if she could find out who I was and turn me in. I did not give up on any of them until I got my sandwich and the guy working there gave me the glass of water in shock. I was going crazy. I was also terrified in the moment I might get caught and get kicked out of school, but not letting someone get the best of me in that moment was a value I had which was more important than my future at that specific time.

After I left, I was feeling terrible. Later that day I was crying as hard as I could. I even called the counselors as the Disabled Programs and Services in tears asking them if anyone reports anything I want to apologize. I hated it, and I hated myself for doing it, but I could truly not stop in the moment. Coming down from that energy of conflict and mania to the depression was going from a state of Rajas to Tamas.

The common thread of all these disorders are the brain states, or executive dysfunction, and what I value when those brain states change, but if I can take a value as not important when it rises in my brain, which means I need to be able to see it clearly, I might be able to control how I feel about that value, or thought, when it rises. If I can control my feelings by seeing my thoughts clearly, with an ability to pause, I would be able to have control over my behavior and actions because, as I stated, it is how we feel about what we think that controls all our actions, and most of us are not even paying attention to all we are thinking even if they do have impulse control. This all takes a pause, but I have to value the pause, and developed my brain to be able to slow down and take a pause with daily meditation. Meditation is the only thing that is getting me to some type of impulse control, which I have genetically lacked my whole life. Today I develop my brain daily to be able just to pause by making a conscious decision to pause in the daily meditation for forty-five minutes.

I have found, for myself, I can have some type of "control" over my actions if I can see what I am thinking clearly and negate the destructive thought instead of valuing it in the current moment, which me valuing a destructive thought is when these conflicts arise. If I have a thought that rises that truly does not serve me, and it is truly not important, especially if it puts my life and future at risk, and if I see it clearly in the moment, I might be able to get from the states of Rajas and Tamas to Sattva by just the negation of the Rajas and Tamas that rises. This can only be done through the clarity of daily meditation. To see the thoughts impinging in all corners of my mind takes a daily practice of meditation. I have to value the meditation.

It is the egotistic and prideful values that are intruding in my psyche. It is how I take creative cruel humor as important that causes lots of my issues in this world. It is the importance of how others perceive me, if they take me as weaker than them or stupider in anyway, then my values surge with my ego. It is the importance of paranoia which makes my heart palpitate and freezes my every move from my anxiety when I would call 911, or the importance of a disturbing thought that did nothing but magnify my depression, which all depressed people find comfort in thoughts and activities that enhance their depression.

These values also manifest in different ways. With my ADHD, when I am trying to pay attention to what I am reading, it is the importance of the next book I'm going to read which keeps me from focusing on the information I need out of the current book I am trying to enjoy. Or with my ADHD, I would be reading, and a word would trigger a different thought, then I would be thinking of all these different things instead of paying attention to the book. I would not know anything that I had just read because I would be focusing and valuing lots of different thoughts, instead of being able to pay attention in any way to the message of the words on the page. Sure, my case is going from one extreme to the other, which might be a bit more complex than some, because my brain does this so quickly and is an organic brain disorder, but this rapidity of constant change has revealed to me what my brain focuses on: nothing but a different value.

This is what happens to all of us whether we have mental illnesses or not. I have noticed we all do this with the similarities I have with others. All humans are controlled by what they value and desire just like the Buddha said. The plus about the Buddha, as opposed to Freud, is the Buddha offered a solution. But they both talk about pleasure and pain, and they both say the most of us are not paying attention to what we are thinking! Yet, it is nothing but what makes us feel good and bad that controls all our actions. We all just want our rewards and pleasures. Not just human life, but all life. This is the Pleasure Principle, and it is an *Ancient Vedic* principle. The Pleasure Principle is how we all learn: rewards and consequences: pleasures and pains.

It was Jeremy Bentham gave this *Ancient Vedic* principle a Western name, and he defines his theory quite well in this thesis: "at any given point we are beings that seek pleasure and avoid pain," but his writing is quite lacking because in his writing he does not give much attention to pain.

Freud gives just as much attention to pain as he does to pleasure, and Freud shows how it determines our behavior. In the *Vedic* scriptures I have seen the best understanding of the Pleasure Principle because the *Vedic* scriptures give just as much attention to pleasure as they do pain. The *Vedic* scriptures also do something most western sciences do not: address the paradoxes that are all throughout this empirical world (Maya) of relativity and duality.

With the *Vedas*, it describes the empirical world as the Maya. The Maya in itself is nothing but an illusion, but the Maya arises from what is true and only true: Brahman, or the One. The Maya itself is nothing but a combination of opposites: hot and cold, bitter and sweet, pleasure and pain, and at the most fundamental level matter and anti-matter. This is why the Pleasure Principle is just as much about pain as it is about pleasure because all duality is the spectrum which rises from the One. This One, or Brahman is non-duality, or Consciousness. It is our ignorance which takes this empirical world (Maya) as dual and relative.

It is acknowledging paradoxes, that Eastern Religions do such as

Vedanta, that I believe modern Western Science could learn a lot from. Paradoxes have been shown to all of us quite clearly in Western Science and the quantum world because the quantum world is nothing but paradoxes: quantum gravity, at what level something becomes quantum, the electromagnetic effect, which is the wave particle duality and is where Heisenberg's Uncertainty Principle was discovered, and is this empirical world digital or continuous digital? All those are observable paradoxes of the quantum world. The justification of paradoxes has been proven to me quite well in these Ancient Scriptures which were the first to acknowledge relativity and duality. If motion and perceptions is relativity; therefore, individual minds and "truths" are relative, and everything has it's opposite, how could there not be paradoxes all around us? Vedanta, like other forms of Hinduism, addresses these paradoxes.

Einstein neglected his own theory, which he won the Nobel Prize for, because it had a paradox: the Electromagnetic Effect, which led to Heisenberg's Uncertainty Principle, but how could any existence of relative truths and duality function without paradoxes? Those two concepts together should let anyone know that the different forms of Hinduism have a better understanding about the "true" function of the empirical world (Maya) than most modern western sciences. Sure, we should continue constantly try to figure out every paradox and every scientific problem! I am all in favor trying to figure out everything in the Maya, but we all need to realize the paradox of Western Science is that every answer just brings about more questions, or as Nisargadatta Maharaj said, "every realization gives new dimensions to conquer." Every time we get any answer in this empirical world (Maya), it does not lead to the end of answers, it only brings about to more and more questions. This is the paradox most Western scientists refuse to acknowledge, and I have proved it to several doctors I have taken classes from!

Einstein said, "God does not play dice" because Heisenberg's Uncertainty Principle violates causality. Einstein denied paradoxes. Vedanta would agree with Einstein on saying God, or Brahman, is quite simple. Brahman is a Non-dual One, that "does not play dice" in anyway, but how Brahman manifests, this Simple Consciousness, is in a very, very complex way because from the One rises relative "truths" and duality. These truths could be nothing but paradoxes at the most fundamental level, and it was Neil Bohr, one of the main proponents of quantum physics in the modern world who said, "Einstein, stop telling God what to do!"

So, the paradox with the Pleasure Principle is that Vedanta acknowledges we are all determined through the rewards of pleasure and pain. This world is just Karma, or causality. With every action, there is an opposite and equal reaction, yet in my life I am the only one that has the power of choice. The rest of the world is determined, and I am supposed to learn from it and accept every piece of it because it is nothing but God. I am here in this ego to grow and learn from my consequences, and in anyone else's life that is what they here for: to learn through consequences. It is only the individual who lives through choice, not because any of us have power of choice, but because there is no other way to live! It is a paradox that we all need to be address! This Ancient Principle goes very well with the *Theory of Evolution* too.

Charles Darwin's *Theory of Evolution* states: "any life that loses its ability to learn and adapt becomes extinct," and how we learn is through rewards and consequences: pleasures and pains. It is nothing but the actions we take that bring about our karma, and we learn from the consequences of our karma. This is what has gotten me to fall in love with *Vedas*. I see so much truth is in them and I have even found the *Theory of Evolution* in such scriptures as the *Chandogya Upanishad*. The *Chandogya Upanishad* talks about all life evolving into all other forms of life, and what I have found with *Vedas* is we either learn or we suffer. It is nothing but ancient scriptures that tell me the same basic conclusion Charles Darwin came to himself.

Once I had the clarity and awareness to see of what the troubles of my brain were through, the reflection of daily meditation, and the Neurological Evaluation I had done at UCSF, I decided to put it into a speech the next day in a class. When I gave this speech,

I asked an active participant in the audience, "What is something important to you?"

"Family." She responded.

"Why?" I asked.

She was in shock! She could not think of why! She had never asked herself why she thought her family was important before. She just always thought they were. This was when I told her, the only reason she takes her family as important is for no other reason than her mind tells her they are important. Most of us can never even look at something as simple as this, and our minds tell all of us what it thinks is the best way for us to survive, family is definitely one of them as a child, so we take it throughout our lives. We all have two problems as rational animals: ignorance and understating. It is right in front of us, but we take it for granted, and most of us are not even paying attention to what we are thinking.

The reason most of us do not see things like this is because most of us aren't even paying attention to the only thing we can see from any angle: our own mind. I had my Hindu guru tell me we all do this. It is not just me, and it is not just the girl I got to participate with me in the speech I gave, who does not look at her mind, but most of us never question our thoughts and the conclusions our minds come too.

The problem is when we look at the world, or try and get information from the world, we are clouded by relativity. We only get a subjective view of the world. But the one thing we can look at from any angle is our own mind. These thoughts are not objective truths, but we can view them in an objective way when we meditate. When I saw the objective view of my own thoughts, I saw how the thoughts themselves, are nothing but thoughts: imagination. The Rajas and Tamas which make up the complications and conflicts of our thoughts, which are nothing but imagination. They are not reality. By sitting in silent meditation watching where my brain states rapidly take me, I was able to get this clarity. My brain would always take me to something it thought was important even when I tried to control where my mind was going at the beginning! I could not! What my mind, or anyone else's mind, does is take what they are shaped to value as important through karma, or causality, so it is those values which control my actions, and everyone's actions. Most of the time it is nothing but our selfishness and our self-seeking desires that we value. We value this selfishness because without desire there is no life. Because without desire there is no action, and without love there is no desire, so again: "life is love and love is life." Nisargadatta Maharaj. We are also always seeking validation of those selfish values and desires through our experiences. It is the egotistic and prideful tendencies within all of us that tells us not to question ourselves and take what we perceive in our daily lives, and the first conclusions we come to, as the truth.

Even with my disorders being so unique, it has been shown to me that I have a lot more in common with people than I ever really thought through the exploration of my own mind in silence. Sure, I have a lot of disorders, but I am like all living things, not just human, but all life on this planet. I want to feel good, and I learn through pleasure and pain. I am also selfish and self-seeking because of that desire to always feel good. It has been shown to me how much I have in common with other people with all kinds of experiences such as the psychology of TV commercials and movies. Through the psychology of both movies and commercials I can see how I am not unique when it comes to other humans because commercials and movies are meant for all of humanity, and I am amazed with how well I relate to them. I find most TV commercials obnoxious, but I also notice they work very well too. TV commercials are meant to stick in our brains.

Wayfair has truly the most annoying commercials, but when I walk down the street, nowhere near a TV, I have had their commercials playing in my head. There was this one Wayfair commercial I thought was so stupid. All it did was repeat the word "better" over and over. The whole commercial was "better, better, better......" Better was basically the only thing it was saying to silly music for 30 seconds or so, yet I was focused on it. My mind was focused on it even when I was not in front of the TV.

I have commercials in my head from childhood. As I stated I think in words, so I memorize things I hear quite easily with my savant skills. I have an OB commercial in my head that popped into one time I was walking down the street with my wife, and we saw a clean tampon on the road. I made her laugh by singing it to her "OB, it's the way you should be. Keep it simple and set yourself free. OB." My wife started laughing really hard and told me how silly I was. I do not have any use for those because I am male, but the song still stuck in my head from the early 80s. I had to have been like 4 years old when I heard the commercial on TV. Years later, at the age of thirty, I can still recall it walking down the street with my wife. My wife found it on YouTube that night, and that made her laugh even harder.

There is only one commercial I thought made no sense whatsoever, and that was about Subaru being about love. I talked to some other people who did not see the point in that one, but it was so ridiculous I still ponder it at times. I also saw how it did not last too long, and you can tell when commercial themes are given up quickly, they do not work for the business.

I have a friend. Probably the only close friend I truly have. He suffers from chronic depression. He refuses to be on medication because of all the commercials he sees that advertise them too. They all have this list of crazy side effects. They list these side effects in a calm and soothing voice to wonderful relaxing music and people finally being able to live their lives again. They show the people who are on that specific drug finally being able to live a happy life. Sure, some people want easy relief as soon as possible, but I hate being on medication because I've been on them for most of my life, and 99.9% of all the psych medications I tried did not work for me either and if they did, they also had side-effects that I had to deal with too. Medications are also ridiculously expensive in America. I, myself, take drug commercials as quite terrible for lots of reasons.

The psoriasis commercials I take as completely evil with the drug Tilts. They have the bride being able to have the father/daughter dance at her wedding because her skin is finally clear. I see how and why they work, but the Tilts commercial, in particular, disgusts me. It is so manipulative, and the people who created it know it. It is why the drug companies play them. These commercials work for some but scare others, and the prices they charge are ridiculous when they do not even pay for the research. They pay for the patent. The government grants pay for the research. Yet, they advertises these commercials and charge ridiculous prices because they know we all relate to having a problem beyond our control, and we all want simple relief. So, I guess, who I am to criticize anything but the price and ridiculous profit they make if they can relieve suffering.

With my friend who struggles with depression I have also noticed the same thing as with myself. He worked for a home improvement store. He worked there, and he hated it. He hated the company. He thought it was a terrible company with what they did to him and their employees. He even blames himself for giving people promotions there. He feels terrible he participated in their corporation. The reason he blames himself, and takes it out on himself, is because he values his dislike for the company so much. He also thinks that because he hates that company, everyone else should as well. It is the self-centered and obsessive focusing on his misery which is the driver of his depression. This is the depression of Tamas. Every chronically depressed person I have met has a self-centered obsession.

I do not think he should blame himself in any way for working for a place which he was making a living at doing the best job he could because I have never seen this man do anything malicious to anyone, yet he blames himself for helping other workers move up the ranks. He takes it as his fault for no other reason than his mind takes it as important. If these values apply to me and they apply to him, then we all have so much in common with our DNA being 99.9% identical as well. What he values does the same thing to him as it does to all of us. They just give us different results, but they are still mental illnesses none the less. They are a mental illness whose disposition is self-centered values.

Movies also show me how much I have in common with people. There have been several movies I have seen that got me to think about myself and how much I have in common with others more than anything else: *Her*, *Three Billboards*, and something I saw just recently *Everything Everywhere All at Once*.

Her was all about love. Joaquin Phoenix plays a tortured character who just wants what we all want: love. This love is pure being characteristic of the Sattva in itself. This emotion of love, how we think of it, and the way it makes us all feel, I thought were exclusive to me. While I was in the audience, I realized, and was overwhelmed by that realization, that everyone in the audience was relating to it. This movie about love was not just for me, it was for all humans, and how we all relate to it. I was not as unique as I thought I was when it came to the needs of romance and love. *Her* was meant for everyone. I had a friend who did not even like it too much who said he related to it.

When I saw *Three Billboards*, it was about what anger does to all of us. Frances McDonald was playing a lady who was a mother. Her child was killed, and the sheriff could not find the killer. McDonald's character took the anger she had over her daughter's death out on the sheriff and everyone in the whole town. I related to this movie as well because I was extremely abused as a child, and I took that anger out on everyone in my life for a long time. I saw in *Three Billboards* how powerless we are over this rage we all can go through. It is not just me who gets into conflicts with other people. It is the whole human race. This passion of anger would be the Rajas.

Sure, I fluctuate quicker, and might be an extreme example of the passion that flickers inside me, but when it comes down to it, I am just like everyone else. I was obsessed with what I thought others were thinking of me, just like everyone else, and I always got some sense of self by what I thought others were thinking of me, just like everyone else does too. We all get this amazing amount of sense of self from what we think others think of us because we are meant to survive together. We are meant live in families, tribes, cities, and civilizations. But because I fluctuate so quickly, I have been able to see how my values change. These values, which change in our brains, affect all of us and control the shifts in all our behaviors. Like I said, each of our minds tells us the best way it thinks we think we can survive. We all just have the same two problems: ignorance and understanding.

An amazing movie that just came out recently is *Everything Everywhere All at Once*. I loved it and I could tell everyone did in the audience too! I could also tell that even the annoying people behind me, who would not shut up through most of movie while it was playing, where reflecting at the same exact parts as I was. We would laugh at the same times, it seemed as though others were shedding tears at the exact times I was, and I started to reflect about my existence and where I was in my life, and I leaned over to my wife and asked her, "is this movie getting you to reflect?"

She responded, "Yes."

I could tell everyone was reflecting because when the whole theater when silent, with a seen of two rocks talking to each other on a cliff looking off a huge Canyon, that they were reflecting with the same questions that were being presented on the screen between these two rocks in a subtitled conversation. They went from laughing extremely loud, to silence! There was no sound from the speakers either! That is how I could tell they were all reflecting! I used the quote from Maya Angelou in the second chapter to prove how much I have in common with everyone despite my rare genetic brain disorder, but we all have desires, we all want to be important, we all question our existence and the point of this ridiculous empirical illusion, which is nothing the concept of this physical world which is called the Maya. It is things like how much I have in common with every single person I meet now that shows me that I am truly not that much different than anyone, and I have this belief reinforced to me over and over when I continue to open my mind. I am not much different than anyone despite my rare brain disorder and crazy background because all life is here to learn. All life suffers, and this pain is one of all our two teachers in the *Vedas*. The other is pleasure.

When people are depressed, they value things which make them more depressed. I have tried killing myself more times than I can count as I stated. A lot of it was for attention, but I even tried to cut my throat one time. That time I meant it. A couple of other times I did too, and I just would not die. One of the things I have noticed since then, is when I was depressed the only thing I held onto in my mind, or valued in anyway, was how terrible I was. I was the greatest most terrible person who ever lived. I valued how terrible I was because I did not have anything else, and being the worst was the only way to be the best at something. I have seen people do this all throughout society. The Punk Rocker and Gangster Rap are the same song to different lyrics and a completely different tune, but we have all been there. That is why those completely different beats are for everyone! Not just me, but everyone!

This depression I went through, and the depression anyone can go through, has its basis in ego. I have seen that in every depressed person I have talked to as well. They all value and take comfort in things, situations, and thoughts that do nothing but enhance and magnify their depression.

Because I had the realization of thoughts being nothing more than just thoughts, and that meant these thoughts were nothing more than just imagination. I saw my problems is that I valued this imagination. This imagination that I valued was what was completely controlling my actions. I have the clarity today to see I could take these thoughts as important or not. Now days, I can value a thought or not value a thought, especially if I can pause and see that thought clearly. I see most of my thoughts are just as important as imagination because these thoughts all have their root in my toxic ego. I do not need to take anything as important or even real because, not just me, but we are all wrong all the time in our relative and dual "truths" that we cling too. I see with myself when my thoughts cause harm to me and others I have been able to negate this imagination. To negating these thoughts, the thoughts of the Rajas and Tamas, would be a good way to address them. Neglecting these thoughts when I meditate allows me to pause and neglect them during the day, which is nothing but one of the mental exercises to rewire my brain's neuropathways.

I can take the power right out of the Rajas and Tamas. Even if a thought is truly important, like the next book I want to read when I am trying to just pay attention to what I am currently reading. Sure, I need to read that next book someday, but at the moment I need to negate any other thoughts except where the words of this specific author are taking me on this very page that I am trying to pay attention too. So, I now have the clarity to see that the next book I need to read is not important in that very moment.

When it comes to what others might be thinking of me, which was what lead to nothing but a self-defensive and aggressive behavior for me for years, I can just pause in the moment and negate them completely. This is how I can solve the problem of my eight different brain states: neglecting the chaos in a daily practice of emptying my mind every morning. But why is my brain so cluttered with chaos?

What is it about all our brains that gets us to focus and dwell on problems to the point where it harms ourselves and others? Some say the nature of man is good. Some say the nature of man is evil. There is a lot of evidence to support both of these claims. What I say is that the nature of man is confusion. Confusion is a problem of the human brain and its intellectual capacities. This confusion of the brain is because of one thing: we cannot understand the best answers out of the options that are in front of us in that current moment. Under-standing these answers is what the brain was created for. Any brain is meant to solve problems, and the human brain has the ability to solve more rational problems than just basic survival. My belief is where all human difficulties truly arise is the ignorance and understanding just as Socrates stated: "no one would knowingly do wrong."

The reason the brain needs to be able to solve problems is because solving problems is our way to the survival of all life, and with evolution we are always growing and adapting. The human brain, and even all animal's brains, are considered plastic. Which means they are meant to constantly grow and adapt with the flux of the Maya: constant changing of a physical world or relativity and duality. All life, be it animal or vegetable, either learns and adapts or it dies.

It is always being focused on the problem which keeps our brains in the problem. The chaos of humanity is not just about ignorance either because there are lots of people who have the answers who do not know how to apply them to their lives. I have had my wife tell me to treat everyone with the same love I treat her. I have had the answer for a while. I did not think this was possible, and I did not think I could implement it. I have now seen if I can do it with her, then I can do it with anyone as long as I value this solution. I work constantly on not valuing the chaos of my pride and ego. Just neglect the pride and ego: Rajas and Tamas, and as Socrates said: "To know is to do." So, when I truly understand something is when I take the right action according to Socrates.

It is amazing how for so much of my life I wanted to solve my problem of fear with something which just brought about more fear. This is why I needed to insult people and feel superior to them. It was about the fear of inferiority. It was about the fear of people, and it just isolated me even more and made me more scared of people.

When people use drugs, gamble, eat too much, and every other self-destructive behavior, we are all just trying to satisfy a feeling of fear with something which brings about more fear. It feels good in the moment, but as the Buddha said is the Second of the Four Noble Truths: "selfish desires are the main cause of all suffering." These desires, in themselves, are nothing but confusion. People cannot see what they are truly doing. Satisfying a desire is also how we all stay alive. We need to eat, and when we eat it feels good. We are all just terrible at seeing how we all chase what feels good to the point where it causes problems to ourselves and others. Why would anyone take any action besides what they think best suites them in the moment? Our minds always tell us what we think is the best thing to do is. Why would our brain do anything else, and as I said most of us are not even aware of our whole minds because most of us do not meditate, especially the way I do in the next chapter on ADHD.

Not being able to implement the solution which is right in front of them is also the main problem I see with the follower of different religions. Most religions tell people the most peaceful and best way to live. It gives them the solution to living their life, but a lot of conflict has risen from every different religion. They have the answers. The answers of religions are nothing but simple logic and common sense. It is the true misunderstanding of their own text, and applying it to their lives, that is their main problem. People do all kinds of terrible things in the name of God. What most people desire who practice religion is the impossible: certainty in an uncertain world.

This desire for the impossibility of this certainty is why their religion does not bring about peace and happiness to them. Their religion only brings about fear. This fear is what the delusion of fundamentalism gives all its followers. The Maya is always uncertain. The plus about Vedanta is it gives certainty in only one place: I am! The only thing that is certain is my existence. Everything else is an inference subject to doubt. This Maya is perfect in one way: It is nothing but my perfect teacher. The *Law of Karma* and the *Theory of Evolution* both tells me the same thing: this empirical world is constantly changing and I either learn or I suffer. This shows the problem of the brain is just as much about understanding as it is ignorance because God would never want us to do anything terrible in any way. We reward and punish ourselves through our own error because we are all hear to learn.

ॐ

I saw for a very long time how I was always stuck in the problem. Especially in the moments when I would lose all control. These situations of complete loss of control were frequent because my brain would value the thoughts which rose, and I was not even paying attention to what I was thinking. It is this same clarity of awareness that has gotten me to deal with my hallucinations. These hallucinations are based in the Tamas. I can now see these hallucinations are just images. Images I do not need to put any value on. I can detach from them and let them go. When I have hallucinations now, I meditate and empty my mind completely, which I will be showing in the chapter on schizophrenia. These hallucinations are more illusions now because I can see they are not reality. I can be in a state where a hallucination is just an illusion, which, either way, it is just a pointless thought, and there does not need to be anything important about the illusion. I have illusions at night sometimes, but they have not bothered me for a while, and I explain how I deal with them in that chapter too. I can see what any thought can be today: pointless imagination.

With this awakening through the combination of meditation and the Neurological Evaluation at UCSF, I now have the ability to put a weight on each of the thoughts I have and see if I should truly value them or not. This has been the best way for me to overcome my eight different brain states is to try and do the mental exercises daily in the next chapter on ADHD and all the following chapters. The Chapter on ADHD in my main daily practice, and I use all the other chapters when necessary, and I can even adapt these exercises when I get more clarity, which is why I am rewriting this book. I have adapted my techniques many, many times. You can also see what works for you and be able to take this and figure out your own mind.

I have been able to take all the power out of the different brain states, get off most medications, and live a productive life. My hope is not for people to get off all psych meds, but to show people how to understand their minds, and work through their own executive brain dysfunction. I have the power to not engage with these different brain states today when I address the brain states through the thinking. I refocus the brain states through Trataka and work on evening the chaos of my mind daily.

Just be aware that I do not identify my True Self, or Atman, which is defined as nothing but consciousness, then when I am identifying my body and mind. My True Self is nothing but my consciousness, as it says in the Rgveda: "The True Self, itself, is that Pure Consciousness, that which nothing can be known in any way, and the same True Self Pure Consciousness, is no different from the Ultimate Principal Brahman, Brahman is the only reality, since it is untinged by difference, the mark of ignorance, and the one thing that cannot be improved upon." In Vedanta the Brahman and Atman are one, but I do have all kinds of issues that I am able to overcome by just being the Witness and addressing the brain states through the redirection of my thinking, which is the single pointed concentration meditation (Trataka) laid out in these scriptures.

Today I can keep my mind from wondering without medication. I am working on the daily negation of all my urges, and I believe it will come with time. Especially when I do nothing but accept the rest of the world as the way it is meant to be. I can feel the energy still being there in my mind and gently say to myself: "who cares?" I just do not need to torture myself by focusing on the value that drives me crazy because, with meditation, I have been able to shift my focus throughout my day no matter what I am doing to get to the next solution clearly. Before I was not even aware of what my mind was focusing on at all. I would just lose all control.

I notice what I am thinking all throughout the day now, and because of this I notice I even have the insanity of an "if/only" situation. I was walking down the street the other day, and a car came close to hitting me. It did not. The car stopped in time. There was also a cop car right there. Then my mind went to the fantasy that the car did hit me. I followed the fantasy to the point where the cop chased the driver down and arrested him. I saw it and pulled my thoughts back from the fantasy. It was a value that did not even happen that was driving me crazy. I was even getting angry over a fantasy. That angry fantasy in itself was the chaos. That Rajas is within us all.

We are all addicted to our fantasies, especially because most of us don't acknowledge that is all, all our minds are: fantasy or imagination. We dwell in them and play the same broken record in our heads. I cannot count how many times I have replayed the situations of what I have said to people which gave me those different brain states. The same situations give me the same thoughts and brain states. These thoughts and brain states are addictive because what we all take as important is what stratifies our selfishness most of the time.

I have found the best way for me to overcome my faults of any kind is to identify them through seeing each thought clearly through meditation, and then I just let them go by not taking them as valuable and not interacting with them. I even am able to shift my focus. If I want to be rid of my character defects, I should not define myself, or identify myself, by them. I should be able to see my character defects as they are there but should not take them as myself or important in any way. These values, and what I have always taken myself to be, are just thoughts. Thoughts do not need to control me, and thoughts do not need to control anyone. We just need see them clearly and let go of the Rajas and Tamas. Just not take them as important. Especially because all thoughts are just imagination. What I have been saying to myself when a thought, or a value, rises in my brain which does not serve me is: "who cares?"

After about a week of having that clarity, I made more progress than I have ever made in such a short amount of time. I have not been to a psych ward or a jail cell in a long time either. It has been over 16 years now since I have been in and institution against my will.

I have been able to just see that anyone else's issues are about them. Realize every single person in this Maya is my perfect teacher. I can pause and see they are having a bad day, or even other complications in their life I do not need to take personally. I can take myself down from my hypomania of my bipolar with the clarity I have gotten by seeing my thoughts clearly, focusing my mind, and detaching from the thinking. I have been able to just remove certain thoughts which do not serve me out of my field of vision. I shift my focus and neglect the thought by saying "who cares?," and when I meditate, I empty my mind completely with just saying those words to any thoughts which rise at all every single morning: "who cares?" is what I say to any thought no matter what it is every morning as practice for forty-five minutes daily.

Anxiety attacks have always been the worst feeling I have ever had; with my new practice, I have been able to focus and see the anxiety attack as just a feeling. A feeling provoked by a thought which does not serve me. When I had these panic attacks in the past, I was someone who would call 911 because they were so scary. Nothing was worse than a panic attack! Truly, nothing! To take this thought as valuable gives me a feeling I do not need to give any credence to. It has been amazing, and it has only come with awareness and the determination to implement this theory, and I have overcome them without medication.

Sri Nisargadatta Maharaja said in the book *I Am That*: "anyone can step over into the solution anytime they like." Progress does not need to be slow and painful. I have always been beaten into the next solution, but now I just do not need to engage with the problem. I can detach from what I once valued.

Seeing what is truly important is something which could help anyone with mental illness, or even the basic problems we all have with our behavior when we have a bad day. That is why these are ancient principles which apply to everyone. My mantra today is "who cares?" We all put so much value on things which cause harm us and others. We value these selfish desires because of our egos. I need to not put a value on my prideful egotistic disposition. I can now just neglect the thoughts of the Rajas and Tamas, or: ~**T**, when I see them clearly. By neglecting the Rajas and Tamas it negates those actions that do not serve me:

((~**T**>~**B**)>~**F**))~**A**.

This way we can open the door to the Sattva. This is what is called in Sanskrit as Viveka and Vairagya, or discrimination and dispassion. The concepts of the *Vedas* have gotten me to ask myself, "Do I want to be a philosopher, or do I want to be a lunatic?" If there is such a thing as the power of choice, it is the ability to see our thoughts clearly, in all areas and corners of our minds, and to be able to neglect any thoughts we have that cause us or others' problems. What we take as important is what controls all our actions, and if most of us are not even paying attention to 90% of our minds most of us do not have much control at all.

If anyone who is reading this thinks they have any power of choice just sit in silence and try to control your mind. Try to keep all thoughts out of your mind for forty-five minutes. You will realize you have no control! Your mind will do whatever it wants, especially when you first start. True power is the power of inaction, or the ability to see your thoughts clearly and then to neglect any thoughts that you have that do not serve you or cause you and others' problems throughout the day. This takes Viveka and Vairagya: discrimination and dispassion. Viveka, or discrimination, is seeing your mind for the imagination it is and being able to look at your mind from any angle. Vairagya, or dispassion, is the ability to say, "who cares?" to any thoughts you have that causes you or others' problems, or to be able to just neglect that thought.

If anyone wants Heaven, Nirvana, Moksha, Salvation, or whatever you want to call it, I have found the only place. It in the here and now. Happiness is nothing but a state of mind, and the mind is nothing but imagination. Just neglect the Rajas and Tamas and let the power of the Sattva shine through. This takes seeing every corner of your mind clearly through daily meditation. This happiness is the essence of Sattva within us all. This is an experiment anyone can do, for as stated in the *Volume One of the Rgveda* "when purified through rays of intelligent discrimination the mind humbly submits to wisdom" through the Viveka and Vairagya.

ॐ ॐ ॐ ॐ

CHAPTER 5

Overcoming ADHD:
Awareness is the Greatest Virtue

MOST OF THE HUMOR THAT makes me laugh is rude clever jokes: dark humor. But as long as there is an aspect of intelligence in the joke, then I can laugh with an innocent one as well. There is a knock, knock joke that is all about Vedanta that was quite harmless, but clever, so it made me do just that:

First, I ask someone who is familiar with Vedanta, "Knock, knock?"

"Who's there?" the subject would respond.

And that is when I would just stand there in silence and not say anything back to them. After a little bit, if they were familiar with Vedanta, they would begin to laugh really hard. The reason why they laugh is when someone is familiar with Vedanta, they would know what I was getting at with the joke. By not responding in anyway, I was telling them without saying anything that, "There is nobody home," or better yet, "Nothing is even there to begin with!"

We are all considered empty in Vedanta at your core to be a Pure Creative Nothingness, but it isn't a "Nothing" that doesn't exist. It is a "Nothing" because there are no words for it. It is non-dual. In modern science we are considered an empirical world of duality and relativity (Maya). Those first concepts or both relativity and duality stem from the *Vedic Scriptures*, and they still hold true to this very day. Relativity means even empirical truth is relative, and with duality, everything that we can detect in this physical world with our senses has an opposite. But what we all are at in our core in Vedanta is a Creative Consciousness, or the Atman. This is something that cannot be expressed in words because it is beyond physical reality. We are all One in this perfect non-duality. It is our misunderstanding and ignorance of misinterpretation which causes all our problems.

This "Nothingness," or Atman, is in our core one with the Brahman and is expressed as the Via Negative in both the East and the West when it comes to metaphysical descriptions of God. The Via Negative is defined as: "it is better to talk about what God is not rather than what God is." This is because God can't be described in words and cannot truly being understood with a relative mind, which we are all stuck with. It has also been by trying to experience God, or the Brahman, I have been able to completely overcome my ADHD.

The meditation in this chapter is my main daily forty-five-minute practice, and necessary for me overcoming all my psych issues throughout the rest of this book. I am not encouraging anyone to get off any psych medications but getting off all these medications is what daily meditation has done it for me. The daily meditation laid out in this chapter is my key practice to even overcoming my psychosis, mania, and autism. Doctors have also come to realize recently that all ADHD is, is a mild form of autism in recent years. If anyone is going overcome anything, they first have to be able to be aware of what that exact issue is and acknowledge it, and if anyone wants more awareness, daily meditation is our best practice to achieve that.

First, I would like to note that none of the pharmaceutical ADHD medications have ever done anything for me whatsoever. In fact, most medications I have tried, and I have tried almost every psychiatric medication and anti-convulsant there is in the PDR, have done nothing for me. Most medications do not work for me because I have this organic brain disorder: heterotopic gray matter, that I talked about in the *Power of Inaction*. I have the aspects of eight disorders with my brain without fitting one stereotype because of the heterotopic gray matter that causes my seizure. I still have simple partial seizures almost every day, and every once in a while, I have a partial complex. These seizures are not dangerous, and I am fully employed today. I was on SSDI for ten years, but the only medication that helps with my seizures now is CBD. I would argue CBD has help mildly with my ADHD as well, but this daily practice has truly made all the difference.

What I am going to be focusing on in this chapter is how anyone with ADHD can overcome their disorder through dedication and a daily practice of meditation. I would not suggest anyone to stop taking any medications. Talk to your doctor about that, but just realize the way I meditated daily, has gotten me off all basically all my psych-medications, and has even helped me over come issues psych medications were not able to do for me, like improve my attention span. The rest of these chapters in this book are about neurological exercise and the neuroplasticity of the human brain.

Neuroplasticity means that we all have the ability develop our minds daily, and nobody is born with an "IQ". This Maya is constantly changing, and our brains are meant to adapt to that change throughout our lives. This "IQ" meaning social and intellectual, not just on a scale from zero to one-hundred-eighty, because "IQ" test are actually a very controversial form of measuring intelligence. But, I have taught myself these concepts through the study of different forms of Hinduism and trial and error of my daily practice of meditation. More specifically, single pointed concentration meditation (Trataka), which I encourage to the whole world to do as well for all our difficulties.

I learned how to read in the year 2007 at the age of 29, as I explained that in the chapter *A Glimmer of Hope*, at the program Linda Mood Bell. Linda Mood Bell was all about the neuroplasticity of the human brain by developing and exercising it specifically for people with learning disabilities. Doing my own research after I learned how to read, I was able to come to the conclusion I can do that with all aspects of my brain that are having issues with the right awareness and daily dedication to develop parts of my mind/brain that is struggling, which is still does daily because this world is constantly changing, which is the key concept of the Maya in Hinduism.

I have every learning disability there is, and I would argue that my dyslexia was not my biggest problem when it came to reading. Sure, not being able to completely interpret symbols easily makes reading very difficult, especially when your d's, p's and b's all look the same. When someone is dyslexic, they have parts of the brain that are over developed, and parts of the brain that are under developed, and those parts of the brain have a hard time communicating with each other. This executive dysfunction causes all kinds of problems when trying to comprehend what is on the page. I also do not think in pictures, which made reading even more difficult I would argue because I had to processes what is on the page. Dyslexia also causes all kinds of issues when writing, but with enough effort that can be overcome as long as anyone is willing to read and write every day, which I have been doing.

My biggest problem I had when it came to reading was paying attention to what I was on the page because of ADHD. When I first started reading, I could spend a lot of time reading without being able to absorb any of the material even after I learned how to pronounce every syllable through the program on Linda Mood Bell. I had read lots of books in my first couple of years of reading with only being able to understand the basic premises that were reiterated over and over throughout the book. This was like worlds that might stand out because they are abnormal to daily language, or just the basic idea of the book.

The problem was that when I read a book, a word on the page might trigger a different thought, so I'd be thinking of something completely different while I was reading the words on the page. When I was finished, I would realize afterwards that I did not grasp much of what was on any of the pages. The biggest problem ADHD is that people with these disorders are not even aware that they are not paying attention. They do not have that capacity to realize they are not paying attention until after the task is over. I am here to testify that with a patient daily dedication it can be overcome without medication through meditation. It is only in this chapter on ADHD, and my chapter with anxiety, that

I am certain with enough dedication anyone can overcome those two issues with this exact meditation. I am wrong all the time too, so this is not medical advice, it is how it worked for me. I also hated being on all those medications. I infer others can benefit psychologically and neurologically with the concepts of these universal spiritual concepts that stem from the *Vedas*. The *Vedas* were meant for more than just me. The *Vedas* were meant for all of humanity.

I no longer suffer from this dilemma of AHAD, at least to the point where I cannot read a book today. Today I can read and comprehend anything in English! I have taken four graduate courses at SFSU in philosophy, and if I can read what I read one semester: Wilfred Sellars, Pseudo-Dionysius, Plotinus, and Robert B. Brandom on empiricism and philosophy of the mind, then I can read anything in English. One of the Doctors in our philosophy department transcribed Wilfred Sellars' lectures into a book, and he said it took him 10 years to completely comprehend Wilfred Sellars. I wrote my final paper refuting Sellars, and the professor who read it said it was well done and grammatically sound. Reading those materials, and writing a good paper, proves to me I can read anything in English today.

That was the most difficult class I have taken so far because of the reading requirements. I did not find one student who completely understood all the authors we read that specific semester. The professor was not that great at explaining anything that he was teaching either. His limitations was the general consensus of my classmates as well. I actually more found the professor's writing on Sellars than his explanations in the classroom.

What I am here to explain to anyone in this chapter is how they can have a better level of concentration without medication no matter who they are! Samadhi is the Sanskrit term that one tries to achieve in Vedanta, and Samadhi is a state of absolute concentration when one realizes the Atman is united with the Brahman within. Samadhi is a state of nothing but Pure Consciousness. All thoughts and vasanas are removed when one is in a state of Samadhi. Samadhi is about the thinning of the mind to that state of absolute awareness. I have not achieved this yet, but it is my goal, and while pursuing this goal it has allowed me to completely overcome my ADHD.

There is a Buddhist chant I like a lot that is relative to this: "Emptiness is nothingness, and nothingness is emptiness." That is what I try to get to when I meditate for that forty-five-minutes each morning. It used to be every night before I got off Saphris. Saphris is a dopamine two receptor site blocker medication, or antipsychotic, which I only take 1/8 of a 5mg tablet if I can't sleep now. The minimum does is 5mg twice a day. I only take Saphris 1/8 of the 5mg tablet so I can sleep now. I don't use it to stabilize my mood and I do not deal with psychotic issues anymore either because of the thinning of my mind.

I have switched to the morning for my daily meditation now. Because I do this forty-five-minutes every morning I have been able to completely overcome my ADHD when it comes to most things. I am still working on my zero-impulse control with my behavior, and I am just now getting to the point where I do not just fire back when I am talking to anyone. Having zero impulse control is what I was tested at in the Neurological Examination at UCSF, and the only thing to improve that in any way has been single pointed concentration meditation (Trataka). I have probably only missed three or four days of meditation within the last six years, and if someone is going to try to overcome their psychological difficulties this way, I would argue they should not even miss that many of their days of their meditation! Meditation is a daily practice, and I cannot tell anyone who is going to meditate to solve neurological issues how important it is to do it daily!

When I first tried meditating, I would sit cross legged in a Zendo on a cushion, but my legs would fall asleep, and my spine would get irritated. So, I switched to a chair, but focusing on my posture drove me crazy as well. I realized my mind was too cluttered to even begin. I could not do sitting in chair either in anyway. These difficulties just mad me give up for years. Especially because I wanted to fit in with the rest of the people meditating. I drove myself crazy even trying! But as Arjuna says to Krishna in the *Gita*, "controlling the mind is like controlling the wind." This is how difficult meditation is even for people without attention issues. The *Gita* is also a book which is meant for everyone because it is a *Vedic Scripture*, but I had to find something that would work for me for all my issues as well. I cannot be that unique, but what I truly had to do was I had to give up on posture and the way I was sitting and just focus on my mind or opening of my Third Eye.

ADHD is usually associated with there not being a high enough dopamine in the brain. This is proven when the people who are suffering are given Ritalin. Ritalin is a medication that is a speed which is proven to boost dopamine in the brain. When people with ADHD are given these medications, in the appropriate doses, which are small, it calms them down and allows them to focus. This is one of the things that proves that ADHD is associated with a lack of dopamine in the brain. But there are other reports of people with ADHD having too much dopamine in the brain. ADHD can even be known to be a type of hyperactivity, or hypomania, and giving a Ritalin would just make it worse because these people with hypomania have too much dopamine in the brain. When people struggle with psychosis, and they are given any type of speed it just makes them more psychotic. With me, I had such a high tolerance to all drugs that Ritalin did nothing after two doses anyways. It was impossible to really tell with me what my issues were when it came to the ADHD.

I believe the problem with my ADHD is too much dopamine because the medications that work best for me block dopamine from getting too high, like Saphris. I have also had problems with psychosis as well. Too much dopamine is known to cause psychosis. This is shown in bipolar type 1, schizophrenia, and schizoaffective disorders, yet because my brain is so complex doctors have speculated that I have either bipolar type 1 or schizoaffective disorder. These dopamine blockers are also medications which have very high seizure rates, like Zyprexa. It is abnormal but dopamine blockers with high seizure rates actually help my seizures. This help and limiting my seizures shows to me that my problem is an over production of dopamine. Zyprexa has a .475% chance of causing a seizure, but it actually made my seizures better. What that means is around four to five people out of every one-thousandth of all people who try Zyprexa will have a seizure. Zyprexa has the highest seizure rate out of any antipsychotic there is, so Paul Garcia MD, was dubious to put me on it, but it actually helped which was nothing he had ever seen before either, even being head of epileptology at UCSF. But I have had lots of atypical reactions to medications my doctors have never seen before as well, which has also made it very difficult to get any treatment, but I am a firm believer in the mental exercises we can all use in such books as the *Bhagavad Gita* and *I Am That* because they are meant for all humanity.

As a child, I hardly slept at all and my mother never really new why. I was just always awake at 4:00 o'clock in the morning watching the test patterns waiting for cartoons. I still do not sleep much more than five hours a night, even on a weekend when I do not have to work. I am not tired at all with this limited sleep. So, I have come to the conclusion is that my ADHD is due to an over production of dopamine, but it could be that my D_2 dopamine receptor cites are too high and the D_1 and D_3 are too low because parts of my brain are underdeveloped as well. Lack of dopamine is a premise of both autism and ADHD, but the point here is that it is really impossible to tell; the best way to overcome this problem, be there too much or too little dopamine, I have found, is this daily dedication of training your brain through the processes of emptying it and single pointed concentration (Trataka). This is a neurological exercise of the brain that anyone can do with a daily dedication to increase their attention span.

It is scientifically proven that meditation increases anyone's capacity for concentration. This proof is what got me to give it a daily effort. I read reports on meditation and concentration, so I thought to myself: "maybe I could try lying down in bed and just putting all my focus on my mind when I meditate?" That is what I did, and it worked! I lied down on my bed and put two pillows under my head.

What I do every morning now when I wake up now is: I prop two pillows under my head and into a comfortable position, then put all my focus on my mind for forty-five minutes on just two words: "I

Am." In my equation $(((T>B)>F)>A)$, or: First I have a thought, then I try to control my brain state through the thought, then the feeling arises from that thought and brain state, and how I feel about those thoughts control my actions. But for the first forty-five-minutes of my day I only do my best to focus on the words: "I Am," or just the T.

As Nisargadatta states "I Am" the only thing we can be certain of. Not being able to do keep my mind focused on the words "I Am" in any way when I first began, showed me how completely powerless I was over my whole life with the equation I have. In fact, everyone who meditates realizes they have no control over their mind in anyway when they begin, at least the ones I have talked to, and I have talked to a lot.

This lack of control over one's thoughts is the consensus I have gotten from everyone who tries single pointed concentration meditation (Trataka). None of us ever had any control over their mind to begin with is what I have gotten from everyone who I have asked who has tried Trataka! Especially the people who try only a once then give up and refused to ever try again because it scares them how little control over their own minds they have. This lack of control just freaks them out, so they refuse to continue. What I have learned through meditation is that it is only by admitting I am completely powerless that I have gotten any control over my mind whatsoever.

When I first started, I would lay down with my white noise app listening to rain drops and I would realize after a little bit I was not concentrating in any way. My mind would just go off in a direction about something that popped into my head. It took me months to even realize this I was not paying attention in any way. Meditation has also shown me everything that is important to me and every motivation I have that truly controls me in every way too. These uncontrolled thoughts were everything that was important to me that my mind was always focused on. I was not even aware of most of what I was thinking was the amazing thing! Having completely zero control over my thoughts and how I felt about those thoughts was mind boggling when we are all living by this illusion of "free will!" This complete lack of control over our thinking is all our insanity!

As was stated in the previous chapter Sigmund Freud said 90% of the mind is subconscious and Descartes said when you meditate you can look at your own mind from any angle. Well, I found both those in the ancient scripture of the *Vedas*, and if anyone wants to see how little control they truly have, be them ADHD or not, sit in silence and try and just keep one thought in your head: "I Am."

Meditation has been shown to me that the only thing I get a universal, panoptical, and panoramic view of is my own mind. That is where the ~**T** comes up is this single pointed concentration meditation (Trataka). The ~ is the negation sign that tells me to gently disregard any thoughts that come up in my mind besides "I Am." All kinds of thoughts would rise when I began, and I told you I am not in a state of Samadhi, so do they still due to this day. I have just lessened them dramatically, and I am always aware of what I am thinking throughout my day today. My mind is much more thinned than it has ever been because I have done this daily for six years, but what I learned to say to myself very gently say to myself in the beginning was: "Who cares?," "I am powerless," or as the Beatles song goes "let it be," then I would gently refocus. This has taught me how to train my brain to pay attention to anything without any medication.

What I try to do in this book is to control my chaotic brain states through single pointed concentration meditation (Trataka): or: **(T>B)**. The more I do it, the easier it gets. This is the neuroplasticity of the brain I was talking about, and we all have, just like the Linda Mood Bell program taught me to do: mental exercises which increasing and develops parts of the brain which are under-developed, but it is a constant daily exercise and definitely not immediate gratification like medication is.

I have learned so much about who I am and what controls me by just lying in and bed trying to focus on what I am at my core: Consciousness! I realized very quickly that I could not just empty my mind out so easily: ~**T**. This daily exercise showed me what my mind always went to that truly control my ego without me even being aware of it. Even if people do not have ADHD, no one else is able to just focus on that Creative Nothingness that we all are at our core without a dedicated daily practice. I had a Buddhist Monk tell me she found it impossible to empty her mind completely and she does not even have eight different brain states that her brain is constantly jumping between. I would argue that if I can do it, so can a Buddhist Monk who tries it this way. She told me the way she meditated, and it was more of just not interacting with her thoughts and letting them pass by. But the way I train my brain is all about rewiring it. It is about directing my reality through my thinking. It is much more of an exercise that I train my mind to do while I relax. That is why it is extremely important to just gently say "who cares?," "I am powerless," or "let it be," and gently redirect your mind without any level of frustration with yourself. So, progress is good, and being gentile with ourselves is extremely important when training our minds. Your reality is nothing but what you perceive, and your mind is nothing but imagination. Our minds being nothing but imagination, is also my main premise for overcoming all my psychological disorders. Today I am almost always aware of where my mind is. When my mind drifts throughout whatever I am doing in a day, I can gently bring it back to the exercise. This awareness is a wonderful and amazing tool for anyone's life!

I would argue that most of what we all do is nothing but repetition. I have been in the rooms of recovery for over twenty-four-years now and I am trying not to cuss as much. I have found it impossible to stop because people who have been in jail cells, on the streets, and do drugs constantly cuss. It is very off putting for lots of people in the average society. I am doing my best to stop. Meditation has shown me that so much of what we do is just doing the same thing we always do. Sit in silence and try and control your mind. You will realize it will always go to the same places, and it will do it without your control especially if you do not meditate. Most of our thoughts being nothing but the same thoughts is scientifically proven too. This is why I constantly neglect so much of my thoughts daily: ~T. Most of all our thinking is just chaos and repetition and needs to just be let go of.

I am now meditating like this every morning. There has also been many times where I have been able to stare directly off into that "Creative Nothingness" that is referred to as the Brahman, and I have noticed my differences in those days too. That Creative Nothingness will be shown to all who try daily. It is amazing that so many of us are so blind to the one thing that we can look at from any angle: our own minds, and behind our minds is that Reality for us all.

Heraclitus, who was an Ancient Greek quite similar to the Buddha, said it best, "You will never in your entire goings find the ends of the soul, though you traveled every path, so deep is its meaning." Sitting in silence; just focusing on your consciousness, will improve your awareness, and awareness is the greatest virtue. Nothing changes for the better without awareness. If we cannot see what our problems are we cannot do anything about them. Because I have gotten this awareness when I am reading anything in English. I am completely aware when my mind drifts from the page on my own, so I gently redirect back to the words. This reading and concentration gets easier and easier, and every once in a while, I continue to notice a quantum jump in my attention span. I no longer worry about not being able to comprehend what is on the pages I am reading because I can understand writers like Wilfred Sellars today and get an A in the class.

So, if you are having problems with ADHD, and medication is not working, or you do not want to be on any narcotics that damage brain tissue like Ritalin, then try daily meditation. I have met doctors who study ADHD who are completely opposed the different forms of Ritalin because they are so harmful, so try meditating every day. Try Trataka in a comfortable position that works for you where you will not fall asleep, but do this experiment with Trataka with a consistent daily dedication. If you do meditate every single day for forty-five minutes, I believe you can overcome your ADHD like I have through Trataka.

Manjushri is the Tibetan God of Wisdom, and He is also the God of Meditation for that very reason. Manjushri will cut through the cloud of fog your mind with the Sword of Fire, which is what allows us to perceive Reality through the state of Samadhi for those who seek it. This is what I am shooting for. I want to be able to achieve a state of Samadhi. My hero is Nisargadatta Maharaj. He has achieved this state of divinity, and with time and dedication anyone can learn to concentrate better and be able to stare off into that Infinite Creative Nothingness. For as is stated in the Mandukya Upanishad "The mind is only brought under control by undepressed effort. It is like emptying the ocean drop by drop with a tip of a blade of kusa grass."

CHAPTER 6

Overcoming PTSD and Anxiety: Thoughts Aren't Facts, They Are Just Imagination

THERE IS A SAYING IN recovery circles of all kinds that "feelings aren't facts." Well, they aren't, but that isn't how I would approach the urges that control my actions. To me it is the thoughts that aren't facts. Thoughts by their very nature are meant to interpret a limited empirical reality (Maya). As a rational animal, humans are blessed with a higher level of cognition, but the problem is most people take what they think and perceive as fact, just like the animal, when what anyone's thinking is, is nothing but imagination.

What all life desires to survive in this empirical world (Maya) is some level of certainty. This desire for certainty was instilled in us through Mother Nature and one of those tools is fear. The instinct of fear let us know when we are in trouble. The problem is, is that the Maya is it is nothing but uncertain. Look at the news. There are people going to the mall and getting killed in America by gun violence daily. Insane and disturbed individuals are just shooting up innocent people all the time in random acts of violence in the United States of America. This gun violence is even happening to children in schools. It is happening to our children all the time, and because it is happening so frequently, that these acts of slaughtering children are no longer the only news story for any particular night! It is disgusting how common it happens! Sudden death by a random gun shooter could happen to anyone in America from just deciding to go to a public place to have a good time or, like I do to, study; therefore, none of us truly knows what is going to happen next be it either good or bad!

Us having this craving for certainty in an uncertain world is clearly where fear and anxiety come from within anyone's psyche, and lot of people suffer from anxiety and panic attacks because of traumatic experiences they have had, which bring about the chemical imbalances in their brains. It is important to note that physical experiences people have alter the chemicals in their brains and cause such things and PTSD, anxiety, and depression. In fact, all mental illness is proven to be caused by two things beyond someone's control: genetics and circumstances, especially in early life, but if you have a problem with anxiety, or even PTSD, like I did; try exploring Eastern Meditation if you want to be able to get over it without chemical treatments: medications. Lots of medications do not work people too, like most did not for me! If a medication works by all means use it, and even use both meditation and medication together for years. This book is all in favor of science, but meditation is what worked best for me over long periods, and this chapter is how I got over my panic attacks and off of anxiety medication.

First, we all need to have a good understanding what truly controls us, which I pointed out in my equation of thinking and human behavior in *The Power of Inaction*: $((T>B)>F)>A$, or I consciously put my thinking before my neurological brain states in single pointed concentration meditation (Trataka), then that leads to my feels, and it is how we all feel about what we think that controls our actions. I will continue to stress that without meditation this is not possible cause I agree with Freud and the Vedas, that for most of us, 90% of our minds are not available to us because most people do not meditate daily.

As I showed you, in *The Power of Inaction* and *Pseudo-Laws and Pseudo-Morals*, the power of choice is more of a necessary illusion for all of us to live by, but if you truly want to see what controls you just sit in silence and try and keep your thoughts (T) focused on the only thing you truly know: "I am." It will show you how truly powerless you are because when you first start this daily mental exercise, your mind will constantly go all over the place. Especially if you have attention issues like ADHD and autism like I do.

What most people take as free will is actually the fact that we all seem to accept the premise we all need to be held accountable for our actions if we have free will or not. This holding ourselves to account by taking responsibility is the best way we can be shaped by our consequences because it gets us to respond to the pain we go through in the best way. The only thing the concept of "choice" really applies to is our egos, but if there is some type of "choice" it would be for each of us to see our thoughts (T) and disregard them if they cause us or another any problems (-T). We need to be able to disregard them because it is how we feel about what we think that controls our actions: ((T>B)>F)>A, and we all have bad thoughts all the time. Just realize that no one does anything except what they think is best at the moment. Why would anyone do anything else? We all think we are much more powerful than we truly are, and the amazing thing is, the only true freedom I have ever gotten from my fears is to acknowledge that "choice" is nothing but a necessary illusion to live by, and that no matter what, in the end, everything is just the way it is supposed to be because this Maya is nothing but my perfect teacher. In the end I am fine either way if my point and purpose in this life is to learn and be a better person. To learn throughout my life is what has given me purpose and make every struggle I go through and overcome as worthwhile. That is the *Law of Karma*: to learn through our consequences.

Once I had the awareness that it was only fear that I was living out of, I was able to ask myself: do I want to live out of fear, or do I want to live out of love? The answer with a sound mind is always love. The problem is the clarity can always be lacking in the moment, especially someone like me who had zero impulse control. Ignorance is the only true evil from what I have seen and what has been shown to me through the greatest philosophers in history such as Socrates, Pseudo-Dionysius, and Nisargadatta Maharaj. As even stated in the *Bible*: "Pride heads the procession" when it comes to the greatest of all sins because pride tells us we are right when we are wrong. We are wrong all the time because we do not know what this Maya holds. To get the right answers to life and to live in peace, we always have to admit when we do not know. That is hard anyone, and this refusal is why pride is the greatest of all sins. Pride is what causes the conflict, difficulty, and chaos between us all.

I was someone who had extreme panic attacks at one time. When I first got sober, because of all the drugs I did, the seizures, and my traumatic life experiences I had, what would happen was from out of nowhere my pulse would start racing, my hands and body would be shaking and sweating, and my face would go completely electrically numb! I did not know why but I felt, for some unknown reason, the world was coming to an end!

I have dealt with basically every mental illness there is with my organic brain disorder, but nothing! absolutely nothing! was worse than a panic attack! I would be calling 911 every single time at the beginning and I did not even know why! Most of the medications they gave me for it did absolutely nothing too!

For lots of other people who they treat anxiety disorders with they give them extremely addictive medications such as Valium, Ativan, Klonopin and other Benzodiazepines. Benzodiazepines are considered the most physically addictive and habit-forming medications there are. My first book *A Vicious Cycle*, is all about a girl who I was in a relationship with who scored all those kinds of drugs from doctors in emergency rooms! These doctors all think they are doing the right thing when they are prescribing them to anyone, but that girl was on a federal list where, if you typed her name into their computer, it would tell them not to give her any drugs, and I still saw doctors give her drugs! Those drugs are all extremely addictive and I am grateful none worked for me more than once because I had an extremely hard time getting sober myself.

I only recommend those Benzodiazepines for people in emergency situations because they are so habit-forming. The problem is lots of doctors had them out like candy, and, like I said, those doctors are just trying to solve a problem and think they are doing the right thing. I had a primary care doctor not too long ago scream at me because I was not willing to take a very hard barbiturate call Primidone. Primidone is an extremely stronger form of Phenobarbital, and people need to realize doctors don't know everything, and lots of medical doctors have no understanding of addiction in anyway. Doctors all have specialties. No one doctor knows everything about all different forms of human medicine. It is an open science that is constantly developing just like all other Western Sciences. I don't either and that is the concept of the Maya: ever answer just brings about another question.

Trying to focus my thoughts for forty-five minutes every day, as I laid out I the chapter on ADHD, has also shown me how to always be aware of what I am thinking in every moment of every day. To be able to look at my whole mind any time I want to is an amazing gift, which got me off the medications they gave me for anxiety too. The ones that worked for my anxiety are not the first ones most doctors try for anxiety but are the ones I would recommend much more than any Benzodiazepine. Blood pressure medications are what worked for my anxiety, and I have seen them work for lots of other people. They do not give a euphoric or high feeling that any Benzodiazepine does and are completely nonaddictive. I would recommend those blood pressure medications for any doctor to prescribe way before they try any Benzodiazepine. The blood pressure medications don't have the risk of addiction and habit-forming chaos that all the Benzodiazepines do.

When I was having a panic attack, I was completely oblivious to what I was thinking because I had never really meditated with any consistency whatsoever. I have noticed sitting in silence, try to empty my mind of all thoughts daily, how ridiculous lots of my thinking is, and how so much of it just needs to be neglected: (-T). Most of my thoughts were not important in anyway. They were even quite ridiculous.

Growing up in a very abusive, an alcoholic household with physical, sexual, and verbal abuse, it what got a lot of my thinking on the wrong track. When I got to the age of thirteen, I snapped because the man I was terrified of had left. I spent my 14th birthday in a psych ward for a whole month. They discharged me without any recommendation, so no one knew what to do with me. It is important to note all those people were just doing what they thought was right.

Then I got shipped too Discovery Academy. Discovery Academy is where my thinking became even more chaotic. My behavior was nothing but defiance and chaos for years because of my childhood household and then Discovery Academy on top of it. I also ending up getting addicted to lots of different street drugs and alcohol once I left Discovery Academy, so those drugs made my seizures much, much worse.

Seizures will also make the chemicals in anyone's brain go crazy, and I was using drugs and have lots of seizures. With all of these uncontrollable circumstances I still believe in the neuroplasticity of the human brain. This was shown to me with time and effort, we can all improve our realities through daily mental exercises and work on controlling our brain states and disorders through our thinking: **(T>B)**. Addressing the brain states through the thinking I believe we can rewire neurons and neuropathways to feel better **(F)**, which will improve our actions: **(A)** this rationalization of feelings only happens through understanding and awareness. That is what silent meditation has done for me through this single pointed concentration meditation (Trataka). The Trataka was outlined in the chapter on ADHD. Meditation gets anyone to focus and cultivate the greatest virtue: awareness. Nothing changes for the better without awareness.

In the *Rgveda*, which is the oldest Hindu scriptures, it says: "The true self itself is the pure consciousness. That which cannot be known in any way, and the same True Self Pure Consciousness, is not different from the Ultimate Principal Brahman. Brahman is the only Reality. Since it is untinged by difference, the mark of ignorance, and the One Thing that cannot be improved upon." At our core is what we all are, in our very nature is a Perfect God Consciousness. This is something that anyone who spends enough time meditating can get in touch with. This is what emptying the mind, and only focusing on "I Am" does for us all. Gets us in contact with what we truly are: Pure God Consciousness. In Vedanta if you can see it, it isn't you! That is why I just disregard my imagination daily: (-T).

The God within me is the same as the God within you, and the same God Consciousness within us all. The Self in me is the Self in you and everyone else; so, the only way for any of us to get in contact with that is to that is to try and empty our minds completely and see any thought as nothing but imagination. When I empty my thoughts, I am neglecting them: (-T). So, it is not that feelings are not fact, it is that thoughts are not fact, and when you have that clarity that just because you think something traumatic, it does not mean it needs to affect you in every way for the rest of your life because what any of us all think is nothing but imagination. We can move forward by letting go of the past and neglecting each thought that arises because "suffering is the price we pay for not letting go." Nisargadatta Maharaj.

When these feelings of anxiety rise now when I am at work, I just see them for what they were: nothing! I just say to myself "I am powerless" or "who cares?" and make a conscious gentle shift to my thinking by neglecting the ridiculous imagination (-T) and shifting my thoughts (T) to the productive work in front of me. Today I can refocus on whatever I want. In the past, when I was having a panic attack, I was barely aware of what I was thinking! Let alone being able to see this empirical world for what it truly is: illusion (Maya). All of my panic attacks are gone, and I do not even use any anxiety medications!

One of the most amazing things I realized in silent meditation is that my mind was always going to what I thought other people were thinking of me. Fear of people was by far my biggest problem, which I have noticed we all have it. I have proven this because, I have never met anyone I could not make angry from what I said to them. It was something I always took as a gift, was to be able to feel superior to anyone in that moment, but it has been my biggest problem my whole life. To insult anyone in an extremely creative way was how I protected myself at Discovery Academy. That is what my first book *A Vicious Cycle* was about trying to overcome. Why would any care what I thought when they did not even know me in any way? I show in *A Vicious Cycle* how I could overcome and upset any stranger with just what I said to them. The fact that we all get this amazing sense of self on what we think others think of us tells me most humans have no desire for truth.

I use human sexuality, and how most humans express theirs, as my main reason and proof to show that most humans care way too much about what others think of them. Human sexuality is also my main argument why most people have no desire for the truth. We all get this amazing sense of self from what we think the world think of us and how we fit into it. I said to a doctor once who specialized in HIV and AIDS once not too long ago: humans have sex .1% of the time for procreation, there are 46 verses in the *Bible* that either mention or approve of polygamy. *Matthew 19:29* is in the *New Testament* and is all about the approval of Polygamy. Polygamy is where human sexuality stems from. Just read the Iliad if any of us want to know where human sexuality truly stems from. Every warrior in that book has multiple wives and each warrior has a male lover. With polygamy naturally comes homosexuality and bisexuality. I would argue most humans are bisexual and we are all too scared to admit it! We are 98.7%, both genetically and behaviorally, like bonobo chimpanzees. Every time a bonobo has a conflict be it male or female, they have sex. I also use the hypersexual female anchors on Fox News to prove my point. It was nothing but my City College Modern Americans Women's History teacher that pointed those women out to me. So what does it mean to be a straight person?

The doctor who studied HIV and AIDS just laughed and agreed with me! He did not think there was anything as a "Straight" person either. If we isolate men with men and women with women, they naturally show homosexual tendencies, yet being gay or bisexual is this terrible thing. Why? Because we are all consumed with what we think the world thinks of us, and I would be putting on sexism as well.

I cannot tell anyone how many times I have a had a gay male friend tell me they had sex with a "straight" married man with children, and then they would ask them the next day when they woke up if they wanted to do it again, and they would say, "I can't. I am straight."

Ok? Whatever that means? Is all I ever thought to myself. But we all get so much of a sense of self on what we think the world thinks of us, and we all want to belong and do things to feel important to the point where it causes us all delusion and anxiety. So just realize, none of us can even prove other people have minds let alone what they are thinking, which I prove in my chapter on schizophrenia later in the book, but the point is to let all anxious and trouble causing thoughts go: (-T), or "who cares?" Negate your thinking daily. Realize your thoughts are only important if you say they are, and most of them are just repetitious conflict we have never let go of. Our thoughts are only important if our minds tell us they are.

I have been on almost every psychiatric drug there has ever been made at one time, and most of them did nothing for me, and when they did, they'd also lower my IQ. I am only on CBD for my epilepsy, but what I have found more beneficial than anything is meditation, for meditation is nothing but the best psychoanalysis anyone can possibly give to themselves. You will see everything that is important to you and that controls you if you just try to keep your mind focused on the only thing any of us can truly know: "I am."

The best speaker I ever heard in a Twelve-Step meeting was a lady who had breast cancer. She just had a double mastectomy, and the one thing she said over and over is, "there are no big deals" which goes very well with "who cares?". A wonderful song which has the premise as my "who cares?" but says it in a gentle voice is *Let It Be*, by the Beatles. Sure, things are important, but there is nothing worth losing our serenity over.

By sitting in silent meditation, I have gotten so much clarity and awareness. I have been able to sift through the chaos of my mind and get in touch with the Perfection within me. That Perfection is within us all. Sat-Chit-Ananda is Being-Consciousness-Bliss in Sanskrit, and that happiness is at our core. We live in an Empirical World of duality. So, with every joyful experience there is pain that can go with that, but the Ananda, or bliss, within is the One Happiness that has no opposite. This happiness can be experienced at any time, and that is who we all are in our very nature. If you want a God which is provable; that can give you peace, then look to the God of the *Rgveda*. That God is within us all, and with a daily practice of meditation you can get in contact with it. You will have all kinds of clarity by sitting in silence. Clarity like you are perfect the way you are because God created you were made this way for a reason: to learn through the shaping of Karma. Acknowledge the paradox that you are perfect the way you are, and when it comes to the mind body duality; there is always room for improvement. You will realize fear is just fear, and as I showed you fear is nothing but the urge to protect someone or something, so the root of fear is nothing but love. That love is the driving force of life within us all that just gets misdirected through our misunderstanding, but anyone can find this happiness by the negation of all thoughts for forty-five minutes daily by saying "who cares?" to any thought which rises. When that happens, we can experience the Sat-Chit-Ananda within us all at any time of the day having no need to panic in anyway.

CHAPTER 7

Overcoming Depression:
Your Perception Is Your Reality

PEOPLE BELIEVE ALL KINDS OF things, so who is to say what is truly true? There is my truth, there is your truth, and then there is the "Truth." I go into this in more detail in the next on schizophrenia and bipolar disorders, but in the scientific reality we live today, this world is all about falsifiability not verifiability. We determine a good theory by using a test at hand which can prove a specific theory false. If the result of the theory stands up to a test which would prove it false, then we validate it by its ability to stand up to the resistance that it was not proven false. A theory not being proven false is basically what falsifiability is, as long as there is an empirical test which could prove it false. If there is not a test that can prove it false, then it is not a modern scientific theory at all. It is just a belief accepted on pure faith, which we all have lots of those: any fundamentalist's interpretation of their scripture. Falsifiability is what Karl Popper clearly proved made Einstein's three theories so perfect with the eclipse of 1919: *The Special Theory of Relativity*, *The General Theory of Relativity*, and *The Electromagnetic Effect*.

With the eclipse of 1919, if those stars that appeared from behind the sun, which were only visible because of that specific eclipse of 1919, were to appear anywhere else on the photo electric plate than where Einstein's mathematical equations predicted that they would be, then something would have wrong with at least one of those theories. Or, if those stars didn't appear exactly where Einstein's theories said they would be, then maybe all three would have been wrong, but they didn't! That eclipse validated both *The Special* and *General Theories of Relativity* and *The Electromagnetic Effect* in one simple test because the stars appeared exactly where Einstein's theories predicted they would on that photoelectric plate! Exactly!

Any Western Scientific theory in modern times is never proven completely true. We only come up with tests to try and prove a good theory false. With the theory of falsifiability, when we come up with issues with a good theory, we just need to find a better theory to replace it. All three of Einstein's theories I mentioned above have problems with them, but they are still our best theories for motion, gravity, and the wave particle duality of light and matter. The paradox of Western Science is every time we get an answer, it does not lead us to the end of questions. Each answer we get just brings about more questions! This is the same concept that the Maya holds in the different forms of Hinduism, especially Vedanta. With all forms of Hinduism, every time there is an answer in this empirical world (Maya), it just leads to more questions. None of us will ever understand everything about the Maya because we are all looking at it through a relative and limited perspective. I got in a debate with this exact topic with a previous Dr of Anthropology I took classes from on Facebook about this, and I pointed out that we are nowhere near *The Theory of Everything*, and every time we get an answer it just leads to more questions! This theory of the Maya holds true to this very day! That professor had nothing to say on the end of our discussion on Facebook!

This assumption that we are stuck in an empirical world of paradoxes (Maya), that every time there is an answer solved, we just get more questions is what clearly proves to me the Maya is "illusory." It is also an empirical world of relativity and duality that makes me take the falsifiability approach to my spiritual beliefs. Falsifiability even shows us that even science uses faith because science constantly makes assumptions, then measures the consequences of those assumptions, which is why we need falsifiability and not verifiability. This using of faith and different perspectives on relativity shows how our own minds are not the "Truth," and no human mind will ever be able to understand the "Truth." We all just have our limited relative perspectives. Some of these perspectives can be quite dark and depressed as well.

So, when it comes to the individual in this Maya, just realize your reality is nothing but your perception. What you, or anyone else, holds as true is nothing but what your own mind to be tells you to be true. We are all wrong all the time when it comes to our judgements in this empirical world. The only thing any of us know for sure is every experience validates one thing and only one thing which can be certain: existence! Or "I Am." It is our beliefs (thoughts), or **T**, which I consciously put before my brain states, **B**, consciously, that influences my feelings and yours, **F**, which controls the results of our actions: **A**. I proved this in *The Power of Inaction*: **((T>B)>F)>A**. So, all our "realities" have to do with the way we think. Shakespeare showed this perfectly in the play *Hamlet* when he had Hamlet say: "there is nothing either good or bad but thinking makes it so. To me it is a prison."

Reality for me was nothing but a prison for the first 28 years of my life or so. I am someone who has tried killing myself more times than I can count. Most of it was for attention. There were times I really tied to kill myself, but I just wouldn't die. I will be talking about how suicidal I was for most of my life in this chapter, and how even as a kid I would dwell in and romanticizes Hamlet's *To Be or Not To Be* soliloquy locked up in Discovery Academy. Just realize I am taking you to the depths of how suicidal and angry for year in my life. This is not me at the current moment, nor do I think I truly had the ability to kill anyone at the time.

I was an extremely emotional and trouble child because of the circumstances I grew up in. Those circumstances were explained in the poetry I opened this book with. The point to that poetry was to explain my mind state as a child and how truly angry and depressed I was. I wrote most of those poems locked up at Discovery Academy. This chapter shows how we are all forced into our different realities, especially through early life experiences. I argue we can all change our thinking with conscious effort. What got me into the solutions of Jnana Yoga was that I realized my reality was nothing but my perception. All our perceptions are nothing but imagination in this "illusion" (Maya), and with seeing this illusion as "nothing either good or bad but thinking makes it so" I no longer live in a prison today.

With the suffering from severe clinical suicidal depression for a large portion of my life, most medications doctors gave to me did absolutely nothing for me in anyway: especially antidepressants. I would argue my depression was considered uncurable at one time. None of the medications they gave me worked in any way, except Prozac. Prozac worked, but not in a good way. Prozac gave me a temporary state of paranoid schizophrenia, which is common with people with some type of Bipolar Type II. I have known to have some symptoms of but not fit the stereotype completely. Just like I don't fit any stereo type completely, but I am more Schizoaffective-Bipolar type as I lay out in the chapter on Schizophrenia.

My depression was untreatable in the modern sense with those chemicals. The first time I tried to kill myself I tried to jump in front of a bus, but I was too drunk to realize I was at the stop sign! Wherever I tell that story all kinds of people burst into laughter, but the first time I got hospitalized for suicide was at the age of 13. I was in the psych-ward for a whole month and spent my 14th birthday there. The hospital let me go without any recommendation because if I was awake, I was completely in tears. I could not do anything except cry if I was awake and I mean that. The second time I spent a month in a psych-ward was the next day after I jumped in front of that bus.

When I jumped in front of that bus, the cops through me in a drug and alcohol detox because I was extremely drunk. The next day I tried to cut my throat with a very cheap blade. I was pulling back and forth on my right jugular vein for a while! It just wouldn't pop! It was a cheap blade disposable razor, so I had to chance, but I was not turned down for SSDI once because of that. That has been a very helpful scar to show others who think about suicide to show them

I have been there too. My suicidal depression was magnified by my addiction, but I can say today I am a very happy person all because my thinking: **T**. My thinking is good today because I now able to "consciously" change the thinking **(T)** through the awareness I have gotten by daily meditation that I outlined in my chapter on ADHD. Now, that I can look at my own mind from any angle at any time, I want to I can make a conscious choice to change my thinking when I see my thoughts not serving me. This is the main gift from daily meditation.

Now that I missed only about three days or so in six years plus of meditation, I have come to completely agree with that premise of Sigmund Freud's subconsciousness. Descartes also believed that our minds are the only thing we can look at from any angle. Descartes' thesis has been proven true for me as well. Being able to look at your mind from any angle and explore your mind on a deeper and deeper level is what Eastern meditation has done for me and can do for anyone. It led me to my two equations of the mind: $((T{>}B){>}F){>}A$ and $(({\sim}T{>}{\sim}B){>}{\sim}F){\sim}A$, or I do my best to make a conscious effort to redirect my thoughts to influence my brain states, leading to my feelings, which controls my actions. I do that while neglecting the imagination that is nonproductive and just cause me or others harm. The trick is even being able to be consciously aware of everything I am thinking all the time. I do this when the average individual isn't even noticing most of what they are thinking because they do not meditate in any way. Let alone daily meditation.

Sure, we all notice about that 10% of our minds that Freud talks about, but I would argue that I am not as different that others as I always thought I was when it comes to what controls me: pleasure and pain. When it comes to such structurally aspects of the human mind 99.9% of all human DNA being identical. Humanity also survives together, so I am really not that much different as it talks about in Vedic scriptures: "the Self in me is the Self in you." This single pointed concentration meditation (Trataka) that I practice in that chapter showed me most of my mind was subconscious. Despite my unique diagnosis, I just want to have a purpose in life like everyone else. Be happy, loved, and accepted. I struggle early in life, which is why I got shipped to Discovery Academy. It was at that school Raul Willard, a "therapist" there, gave me the true meaning of the Shakespearian soliloquy of: *To Be or Not To Be*, or as Raul told me "to live or not to live."

Even just having a third-grade reading level for most of my life I spend hours going over that soliloquy romanticizing and magnifying Hamlet's misery in my mind as well. What Hamlet described about suicide was exactly how I felt when I pondered the verbiage of his poetry. I related with every single word of this poem as a fourteen-year-old kid! Exploring dark, dark writings in history is what got me to write my poetry. It also shows me looking back how each of us feel in that suicidal state of mind.

I saw Hamlet was trapped in the same dilemma I was. Hamlet wanted to kill his uncle. I had someone I saw shipped away for threating to kill, and I wanted to kill myself just like Hamlet. This soliloquy describes Hamlet as extremely depressed with his circumstances and the twisted perversion of his "prison" of his mind. This was the essence of my tortured mind as well. The first time truly understood those words my mind pulled me into the third act as I sifted through Hamlet's "insanity."

Act Three, Scene One is the most famous *Hamlet* scene. It is in this act that Hamlet's intelligence shines, and like most geniuses, his "sanity" questioned. All of the circumstances Hamlet has gone through cause conflict, and the definition of a Shakespearean tragedy unfolds. In a Shakespearean tragedy it is important that everyone dies in the end. Death is what Shakespeare meant when he wrote tragedies, and I believed for years that my own death was the only true way for there to be any peace for myself at all. At least I told myself these grandiose delusions that only perpetuated my own torcher.

My actions were nothing but chaos as a kid, and I could only dream that they were as well thought out as Hamlet's because he was one of the true geniuses in English Literature. Hamlet is enraged with his uncle Claudius for lots of reason. The main reason is that Claudius killed Hamlet's father with poison. By Claudius killing Hamlet's father, he was able to marry Hamlet's mother. Claudius does this to become King himself. This is disturbing to anyone, especially a son. Claudius robs Hamlet of all of his happiness, and even a chance to be King himself one day! Hamlet seems at times as though he will lose all control over his actions because of his uncle, but the reason why anyone would not take Hamlet as mad is shown through all of the control Hamlet has over himself. Hamlet is very thoughtful and does nothing carelessly. He is cautious and even sagacious, especially in Act Three, Scene One.

Hamlet first recites words that would make anyone convinced that the person was mad. These words were the same words my mind focused on as a child. We are all created with both anger and the hope of love in our hearts for others, but only the sane ones will choose what Hamlet and I chose because we could see this world for what it truly was. This is what my mind told me at the time!

Hamlet might have had some type of psychosis from all of the traumatic experiences that he has gone through. I had a reason for what I wanted to do too. It wasn't just that these feelings and emotions I had come out of nowhere, but because I was locked up as though I was the one who did something wrong? When I was nothing but a product of my childhood abuse! I had a speculation that Hamlet had some type of thought disorder too because Hamlet senior comes to Hamlet as a ghost to tell him what Claudius did? Hamlet's father being murdered, and his Crown stolen from him, was why Hamlet needed to carry out revenge. Revenge was what I wanted as a child too! Revenge was what I craved! To say I was crazy would be to say I had no reason for wanting to kill! I had a reason just like Hamlet! Was my revenge philosophical, or was it insanity? Mine was carefully thought out too, just like Hamlet's, so, if it was a rational thought, how could anyone say that the sound thoughts of homicide and suicide are "insanity?"

My crazy mind took it that it was the rationality of this soliloquy that proved Hamlet was not insane. This soliloquy showed me how screwed up this world truly was. It was also the way Shakespeare's genius spoke to my mind which proved I was the "sane" one as well. There's clarity in all Hamlet's words. Hamlet has been betrayed by so many people, and it is this betrayal that sparks this vicious behavior. That betrayal was the same betrayal I had as a child. I hated the people who raised me for what they did! My rage was calculated and cultivated for years underneath his rule! Now I was the one who was locked up, and he was able to roam the world without any consequences!

Hamlet's cautious reactions to every situation is shown when Shakespeare writes, "there is a method to this madness." Those are words that Polonius states, so even Polonius is not completely fooled by Hamlet. Polonius is Claudius' advisor. Polonius is the panderer who is trying to help Claudius achieve what he wants. It is this same pandering that got them all to take that man's side and lock me up is where my mind romantically went as a child!

Hamlet obviously acts out the obsession, but Polonius is convinced that the cause of Hamlet's obtuse behavior is his love for Ophelia. Ophelia is the beautiful daughter of Polonius, and Polonius is sure love has been denied by her. Even the Queen is hoping this is the case. For if it is, and Ophelia reciprocates her affections to Hamlet, all will be well. None of these people know the truth about what Hamlet knows. None of these people knew revenge is the only thing on both our minds! Just like Hamlet, no one knew my truth either! My mother did in some way, but I was the one locked up at Discovery Academy! That place me so much worse than I already was too!

This seen is an empty dark stage with hard wood floors. There are lights, but they are focused directly on the center of the stage so that darkness drowns out everything else. There are two large red curtains that are parted in the middle. The parts are held back with golden rope. There is a large black curtain behind the two red ones. The Queen is wearing a long dark blue dress. Claudius is wearing an amber robe with his golden crown, and Polonius is standing to his left dressed in black. That dark room where all the counselors at Discovery Academy just had me stand against a wall until the punishment was over was a straitjacket of the mind that school put me in. That Dark Room that I was locked in was actually bright white walls with a green carpet right next to the gym. It was only four feet wide and twenty feet deep. The gym separated the Girls Dorm Room from Unit One. Unit One is where they kept me isolated for basically a year because of the anger I showed. Dr. Thorn, who cussed me out for cutting on myself, told my mother I would be the next Charles Mason because of how much I rebelled! Yet, in this Scene, after they are all done conversing about Hamlet, and what to do about his mental dilemma, all of them exit the stage. All except Polonius, Claudius, and Ophelia. Polonius and Claudius hide behind a curtain when Hamlet comes into the room to watch what happens. The only part of Polonius and Claudius that the audience can see are their faces. They both think that Hamlet does not know they are there watching him. Hamlet takes center stage along with the spotlight. Ophelia is on the far right of the stage in a peach-colored dress that has white laces. Both Claudius and Polonius are listening to try and see all of Hamlet's true opinions and motivations. Even with this trick they are all trying to play on Hamlet, it is them who are deceived.

As Hamlet utters the famous lines, "To be or not to be," Hamlet's discourse about suicide is a romantic argument. It is: should I or should I not kill myself? "Killing myself," as I said Raul Willard told me, was what I thought was the only true choice anyone who can see this world clearly would take. That was the choice I felt they kept me from achieving at Discovery Academy, and Hamlet was arguing this out loud. I always have talking to myself out loud as well just to processes my thoughts, so it did not seem strange to me, and just like I muttered "should I kill myself or not?" So, is homicide and suicide philosophically justified or just plain "insanity?" Was the question I struggle with for years.

In lines 64 through 73 are the bluntest descriptions of suicide, and the hopelessness of Hamlet's words weighs everyone down. "The heart-ache and the thousand natural shocks that flesh is heir to." (Lines: 70-71) Hamlet is talking about everyone's life. He is telling those watching that every person feels this pain. Life is difficult, there is no way out, and it is difficult not just for him but everyone. The whole world was the problem for me at the time too, so it was mankind as a whole! Anything and everything is just misery to the ones who are truly able see everything clearly! That is what the school Discovery Academy really drilled into my head even for years after I left!

Then in line 72 it goes to one of the most sought-after questions of man. Is there anything after death, and if so, what? "To die, to sleep- perchance to dream?" It is in that dream which Hamlet is implying life after death. Everyone in the audience knows this is the need for God and every single religion. Hamlet is clearly stating it is not this life, but what comes after that truly matters. Hamlet and I were both consumed with this fear either way. All the many times that I had ever thought about truly killing myself it was what was after this life that kept me here! Was there misery waiting for me there too! Either burning in Hell, or the fear of not existing at all! Neither was a good outcome in this prison of my mind!

Hamlet goes on to give amazing detail about all of the troubles that everyone has to face. He is proving to the watcher everyone goes through hell. Hell for both me and Hamlet at those times was here on earth. The only reason one would ever put up with this life is because what is next! That is what Hamlet means when he states, "the undiscovered country" (line 87). There were only wishful fools that hoped of something better beyond this empirical hell we were all trapped is where my mind always took me when it came to God because of the fundamentalists in Utah! That was why people believe in "Heaven." They all just needed something which told them there is a reward for doing right when none of us know for sure! They were the ones that truly seemed nuts to me! So, does anything truly matter? Humanity just seemed to convince themselves something did because we needed to believe we are important! That there is a purpose to all the different belief systems, and in the end, if Hamlet kills himself or not, he is completely damned in either way! Just like I was! This is the convincing conclusion, and Hamlet knows it! This was also the only way I saw the world as well! We were both right is where my mind took me for years! Life was torture!

When Hamlet points out Ophelia to the crowd the lights on the stage brighten to where she stands. It is this that brings Ophelia and her actions into the scene. Ophelia would be staring softly with her head tilted down in the opposite direction as Hamlet, as to pretend that she is only thinking of him. She is even trying to hide the fact that she knows he is there, even though she has herd everything. She then notices him and comes forth to spark the conversation.

I could only dream of having love. I wanted just to be loved as a kid just like any other. It was nothing but fear of every single person that was around me that kept me from getting loved in any way, because as a child I was abused child locked up in Discovery Academy I was just as angry as Hamlet! I felt at that time in my life love was beyond anything God would give me. In truth, God doesn't give love to anyone, for how can any of us truly prove there is a God is where my mind went being trapped and punished daily by fundamentalists? They also sent me there for a cure! At the time I was nothing but a pessimist because of my circumstances! I took life as just a deceptional trick from the Kings of every society. Just like Claudius, we were all just thrown into Discovery Academy because none of our parents knew what to do with us! Discovery Academy was all for nothing but control, so how could any even have love? Yet, it is when Ophelia brings her innocent demeanor into play that Hamlet slaps her with cold words.

There is a look of shock on Ophelia's face when Hamlet asks her if she is honest and fair. In lines 113 through 163 Hamlet is yelling as loud as he can at her. He is putting all of his anger onto the stage, and even though he is looking at Ophelia he is also indirectly talking to Polonius and Claudius. Hamlet calls her out on the trick she is playing. He knows they have all been there the whole time. Hamlet makes a direct statement to Polonius letting him know he is a fool and telling Polonius to be a fool only in his own household. Hamlet tells Ophelia she needs to purify herself by going to a nunnery. He is telling her she is a sinful slut, for the trick she is trying to play. She needs to get rid of her sins because she is nothing but a slut!

Lines 160 and 161 Hamlet raises his voice as loud as he can and says, "Those that are married already, all but one shall live!" It is in this statement that he is telling his uncle Claudius that he is going to kill him! He says it to Ophelia, yet it is truly directed towards Claudius! After Hamlet yells all of this vitriol, he runs off of the stage! I had a man I wanted to kill as well as a kid! Killing him was why Hamlet's anger spoke so clearly to me! I was a teenager, but I comprehended every single word Hamlet spoke! The only thing I read perfectly was Hamlet soliloquy because of his anger and pessimism! It took me hours of reading it and pondering it, but there was nothing to do the whole time I was at Discovery Academy except isolate romanticize my misery! That school trained my mind to think in a suicidal depression for years afterwards!

After Hamlet exits, Polonius and Claudius come out from behind the curtain. They run up to try and comfort Ophelia, for they just witnessed the conflict as well. They are shaken just as bad as she is. In lines 163 through 175 Ophelia talks with anguish, and on the brink of tears. She painfully remembers the love they had, and that for some reason it is gone. Ophelia is very confused and scared. The Line "O, woe is me" (line 174) reveals her agony.

I picked Shakespeare's *Hamlet* to write about to show anyone the type of depression I felt as a kid because of my early life experiences. As I pointed out in *Pseudo-Laws and Pseudo-Morals*, there is no need to resent anyone when you take the power of choice out of that person's hands and realize we all have the same two issues: ignorance and understanding. If you sit in silence your reality will be shown to you by your thinking. If you sit in silence, you will realize you have the ability to change your reality because you will see how ridiculous your own thinking is. I showed how grandiose and angry as was above as a little kid, but because I can see my mind from any angle today, I can make that conscious choice to put my thinking before my brain states to control my feelings and actions: $((T>B)>F)>A$ in my symbolic equation.

When I first started to meditate, I was quite overwhelmed with how loud the chatter in my mind was. In fact, most of my life, before I meditated, I would listen to music on headphones playing them as loud as I could. I'd even walk around singing as loud as I could, in large-populated cities, to escape my mind that was screaming at me! It was as though nobody was around, and for me, in those moments, nobody was. I believed I was truly unaware of why I needed to walk around singing so loud. Looking back, I am sure it was obnoxious to anyone around me, but I was completely oblivious to everyone. I see now how I was doing this to drown out the noise of my loud obnoxious mind that was always screaming at me telling me how worthless I was. My mind was screaming at me, and I wasn't listening to 90% of it, which was why I was so angry and chaotic for so long. My mind was always telling me how worthless both me and the world was. This music was how they finally got me to behave at Discovery Academy. I did not respond to any punishment they gave me in anyway. It is why I would listen to loud music on drugs too. I Just wanted to block out my reality! I just wanted an escape the prison of my mind!

At Discovery Academy they would say, "Justin that is a demerit."

I would respond, "F- you, give me another!"

Then they would say, "Let's go Unit One." If anyone got sent to Unit One, they would automatically get ten demerits. I demerit was 25 minutes standing up against a wall, if we moved, we had to start over. With my oppositional defiance disorder, and I proved to them all they could not control me with punishment. I had the head of the female consolers in tears in the front office screaming, "I'm not fat!!" I had one of the head of the male consolers head butt me in the face because he had me pinned up against a wall in Unit One, so I asked him, "Common Rich? You want a kiss?", and I reached out to smooch him, and pop! Right in the face. There was blood dripping down my noise. Rich dropped me to the ground because he wanted to beat me up, but he knew he could not because he was the adult paid to watch me, and I screamed out, "Come back I love you!" as he walked away shaking!

That school is where my depression and oppositional defiance disorders skyrocketed! When Discovery Academy offered me music, I shaped right up. I was not any better in any way. They just had to give me something I desired. I always desired to be in another state of mind, which is what the music did for me. Getting into another state of mind is why I got into drugs and alcohol later in my life as well, but if I focused on the lyrics of a song, my reality was always more pleasant because my mind was preoccupied with the lyrics.

Sure, lots of the lyrics did things like magnify depression. There were songs about suicide with Metallica's *Fade to Black*, or songs about isolation like *I Am a Rock*, *The Sound of Silence*, and *The Boxer*, by Simon and Garfunkel. I always tell people it is amazing how much Paul Simons lyrics will magnify I child's suicidal depression: "I have no need of friendship, friendship causing pain. It is laughter and it is loving I distain." "Hello darkness my old friend." "When I left my home and family, I was no more than a boy. In the company of strangers. In the quite of the railway station running scared." "I am leaving. I am Leaving, but the fighter still remains." Those three songs especially magnified my depression for years. Just like Hamlet's soliloquy did.

When people that are depressed, they find comfort in things enhance and magnify their depression. Discovery Academy was just a place to put me because there were no other options. I see that today. None of their parents wanted their kids going to jail either or ending up in a worse place, so when I saw things clearly, and I work out all my resentments through single points concentration meditation (Trataka), is when I was able to realize there is no one for me to hate or resent in this life in anyway. If I want perfection, it is only through taking this world as being my perfect teacher. I either learn or I suffer, and we all have the same two problems: ignorance and understanding. I am still ignorant to this day because "every realization gives new dimensions to conquer" as Nisargadatta Maharaj would say when it comes to the Maya.

Anyone can apply lessons they learn from meditation into every aspect of our lives. One of the things I have become aware of through

Trataka is that I was always saying things to myself like, "I want to die." "I hate this." "I'm such a f--- up." I was also seeing constantly what was wrong with the world in a very derogatory and creative way as expressed above. It was constant, and for most of my life, I was completely unaware of it because I did not meditate. My mind was nothing but a dark cloud of delusion. By becoming more aware of my thinking, I could begin to contemplate that perhaps these thoughts are not really what I want. So, we all need to realize what Hamlet said when he said "There is nothing either good or bad but thinking make is so."

Today I have been able to make a conscious effort to change my thinking. I try to focus on just one saying: "I Am," which is the only thing any of us truly know. I will prove "I am" is the only thing indubitable in the chapter on schizophrenia later, but when any other thoughts rise in my mind when I meditate, I say to myself: "Who cares?" (-T) Then I try to slowly and gently stop thinking and get in touch with my nothing but my Consciousness. All of that was outlined on the chapter on ADHD, but I am not that good at dropping my mind completely still to this day. Some days, with my organic brain states shifting with thoughts, it is much more difficult than others, but I continue to make progress and develop the neurotransmitters in my brain by addressing the thinking: **T**. The amazing thing is how powerless I am over my own mind. I have heard from lots of people that they refuse to meditate because it bothers them how they have no control over what they are thinking in anyway. Anyone who begins meditation, it will be shown to them how truly powerless we all are.

One day when I realized the entire negative self-talk that was filling my mind, I began to tell myself: maybe I should replace those negative thoughts with more positive thoughts? That day forward I started replacing every negative thought with the words "I love you." I just thought of my wife and said to myself every time I was to say, "I want to die, or f--- this and f--- that." I should just think of my wife and said, "I love you." It is simple and it worked. I am no longer a pessimist. I do not struggle with suicidal depression in an extremely long time. What I did is I took one thought: **T**, and didn't neglect it, or ~**T**, I just replaced it with another **T**! It was a negative thought that needed to be replaced with a positive thought, so I was just replacing one **T1** for another **T2**.

It is important not to try to exorcise thoughts from your mind or get angry with yourself if you are thinking a certain way. Just acknowledge it, and then replace it, and it is not about denial or ignoring any thoughts either. It is also an extremely slow process, which is why I do it daily. It will make you go even more nuts if you get frustrated with yourself or expect immediate gratification. If any of us have a thought that we value and causes us problems, then we can gently say "who cares?", or as the Beatles song goes, "Let it be." Let it be I have noticed is much gentler for most people. If we are constantly thinking negative thoughts, we should take a conscious effort to reshape and redirect our thinking to positive thoughts. Even Hamlet himself acknowledge all our reality is nothing but our thinking! When we can replace one **T1** with **T2**, then instead of getting the wrong actions: **A1**, we get a better outcome because we get a whole new thought to redirect our daily thinking: **((T2>B2)>F2)>A2**!

These days I work constantly on replacing every negative thought with a positive thought. It is slow but gets easier and easier the more I do it. From what I have noticed now I do it automatically. Sure, everyone once is a while I catch myself saying the negative thought, but I just gently say to myself, "I love you." Never get angry or frustrated every time you have a negative thought either. I also say such words as Ahimsa, which is a Sanskrit word that means cause no harm. I have found the pleasure of life today in every experience be it good or bad cause now I have realized life is about learning.

Both the *Law of Karma* and the *Theory of Evolution* tells us: this empirical world (Maya) is constantly changing, and we either learn or we suffer. So, we will all always make mistakes as long our Souls are trapped in our bodies because of the ignorance and understanding that we all suffer from. We are all just here to learn. This is also why I no longer recent anyone from my childhood and I was the one telling my father I loved him when he was dying. If anyone is ever wondering what to do in any situation it tells us in such prayers as the *Prayer of Saint Francis*: "to understand is to be understood," and "to forgive is to be forgiven." So, there is no reason to hate anyone. Just realize the Self in me is the Self in you, and when we take the power of choice out of anyone's hand there is nothing to recent. God does not punish us. We reward and punish ourselves through our Karma and when can always be grateful when we can learn.

I saw a video with a little girl. She was quite my teacher. She had Fibrodysplasia Ossificans Progressiva, or FOP. It is extremely painful medical disorder. Anyone who gets it dies every young. What happens is all the muscle tissue in the body slowly calcifies over their life, so their muscle tissue turns to bone, and they slowly freeze. This little girl was explaining how grateful she is that she still gets to wash the dishes. Doing the dishes has never been one of the highlights of my day, so I thought to myself, if she can shape her mind to gratitude for that, I am sure I can too for much more that I have been given in this life. If you want to be happy, change your thinking to gratitude, but you cannot do it without awareness, so daily meditation in necessary.

Someone told me once he prays for anyone that he has a resentment for. He said he did not know why, but when he did his anger went away. I told him it is because you are taking a negative thought and replacing it with a positive thought. That is why. Being grateful and redirecting our realities helps all of us repair our brains from our troubled and dysfunctional circumstances so our minds can function properly. It is all shaping the neurotransmitters into a positive light, which all of humanity needs at times. I had people tell me I was one of the angriest people they had ever met when I was anywhere from the ages of twelve to twenty-eight. I have changed that completely today and am off most medications, and a functioning member of society. I was someone who had been hospitalized for trying to killing myself more times than I can count but am doing extremely well these days. I don't feel suicidal at all anymore. Just remember our realities are nothing but what we perceive, and our minds are nothing but imagination;

so, "there is nothing either good or bad, but thinking makes it so" as Shakespeare proved to everyone in history. Just meditate daily to get the awareness because the only thing anyone can get a panoptical, panoramic, and universal view of is their own relative mind, then take any bad **T1** and replace it with a positive **T2**.

CHAPTER 8

Overcoming Schizophrenia and Bipolar: Looking is more fundamental in the Space of Imagination

HUMANS HAVE THE GREATEST ABILITY of all living creatures on earth to get to some type of knowledge out of our experience in the empirical world (Maya). We communicate the conclusions of reality that we have come to each other through the expression of semantics. Other animals do not have this capacity to comprehend "reality" to the extent we can, nor can they communicate it to one another. We are never able to get to a complete knowledge of "reality" because of our limited perspectives based on our relative experiences therefore, some type of skepticism is required when exploring the empirical world (Maya). What we need to be able to do is always allow for correction in our error of different thoughts through falsification, and in an empirical world (Maya) of the reality of falsification, it means we never completely get to the truth about the empirical world (Maya) that is around us, but we can get a better and better understanding of this empirical world (Maya) through the gift that humans have been given of psychological nominalism: the attempt to express reality through semantics, because all we can do is attempt to express this Maya. This means that with the gift that we humans have according to Wilfred Sellars' "Space of Reasons" the most we all can truly do is look.

Wilfred Sellars wrote how seeing is more fundamental for humans than looking, but Sellars says when we see, there is a chance we can always be wrong. I would argue that Sellars cannot have it both ways. One cannot say that seeing is more fundamental towards knowledge, then leave the chance that we can always be wrong with a self-correcting falsification if we refuse to look. If we can always be wrong, and we know that through our individual experiences, then it means in order to get closer to the absolute truth, using the Space of Reasons, looking is more fundamental to getting answers than seeing because looking in its very essence allows for the falsification and self-correcting aspects of knowledge. I would argue that for basic survival seeing is more fundamental. This is proven to me because seeing is only what animals do, but if it is to get answers of reality that are desired throughout the Maya, then looking is the gift that humans, the rational animals, have. With looking, all we have is what we infer, and if we are going to be honest with ourselves in the universe of falsification, then inference is all we truly have being that human reality is in the Space of Reasons for every question except one: do I exist? Because the only thing we do when we look and come to conclusions about this Maya is infer.

Looking means we do not completely have the answers, and we can admit that whatever is in front of us we could be mistaken about. I define myself as an inferentialist, and Robert B. Brandom in *Articulating Reasons an Introduction to Inferentialism* explicates perfectly what inferentialists do: "Inferentialists seek to define representational properties in terms of inferential ones, which must accordingly be capable of being understood antecedently. They start with a notion of content to determine what is a reason for what and understand truth and representation as features of ideas that are not only manifested in but actually consist in their role in reasoning" (Brandom P524). I appreciate how Brandom puts philosophers into two categories. Instead of empiricists and rationalists, Brandom describes them as representationalists and inferentialists (Brandom P523). For I, myself, take "truth and representation as features of ideas" just like Brandom states. All I have myself is what I infer about reality, and that is why I hold myself to the class of an inferentialist.

In *Empiricism and Philosophy of the Mind*, Wilfred Sellars explicates how looking is parasitic on seeing. Sellars tells how when someone sees something, like a red triangle, then they are endorsing that object (Sellars 39). To see something means that is how that object is, if and only if, it is how that object is in normal circumstances, and when someone is seeing it, then they are endorsing it according to Sellars because he writes, "For to say that a certain experience is a *seeing that* something is the cause, is to do more than describe the experience. It is to characterize it as, so to speak, making an assertion or claim, and – which is the point I wish to stress – to *endorse* that claim" (Sellars P39).

I, myself, have a problem with endorsements and claims of certainty. I have found that people, in their everyday experiences are always endorsing all their experiences, and they take it as true for no other reason than it is their experience. Most people, from what I have seen, have no ability to question themselves, and most people, even philosophers, are not after the truth. What most people want is the impossible: certainty in an uncertain world, and people take instances that are only supposed to be lookings and take them as seeings for no other reason than they want to know that what they believe is true. I would say that people tell themselves they want the truth all the time, but they are just not honest with themselves. If the truth is what is desired in this Maya of falsification, then the most we can say in any circumstance is this is how something appears to us now, especially if we can always be wrong as Sellars states. This is how this object looks to me in this circumstance, for I can never truly know if my circumstances are ever normal.

Sellars in his *Section III, The Logic of Lookings*, gives a perfect example of how we can always be wrong. Sellars gives a thought experiment of a gentleman named John on pages 37 through 46. John works in a necktie shop, and his whole life he thought he was seeing the ties for their true color. He had always assumed that his experiences where the experiences of seeing these ties were done in normal conditions, then one day someone was able to show him when you take the tie outside into normal daylight the color of the ties are different than the light that John had always been looking at them in; therefore, the conditions that he has always been seeing the ties in were not normal conditions. John was looking at the ties under an electric lighting. This changed all the colors of the ties. When John had this awareness, he was then able to correct the assumptions that he had always been making about the colors of the ties.

What I would say is that everyone always thinks that the conditions they experience things in, and the conclusions they come to in those conditions, are that of normal conditions until they are shown otherwise. We all function off the assumption that our experiences are the true experiences of normal conditions because of our necessary instincts for survival. We need to be able to constantly respond to our current conditions in order to stay alive, and that is what our senses allow us to do, but the only people that are ever able to get to some type of correction of their false beliefs are the ones that allow for the self-correction through doubt. The reason why we always think our assumptions are true until shown otherwise, is because that is what animals do in order to survive. It is important to note too that life is about survival in every instance of our lives, and we are nothing but rational animals. Sellars shows how when John is exposed to seeing the ties in the sunlight that what he perceived was wrong. John can make a correction, but John also has a difficult time doing this. Now John when he is in the store needs to pause when explaining the colors of the ties to the customers. John can express to the people he is selling the ties to that the colors they see in this electric light are not the colors of the ties in normal conditions. There is a doubt which rises in John's mind whenever he is explaining the colors of the ties to people.

Descartes was one of the first Western Philosophers that allowed for some type of skepticism in the modern sense, and Descartes, and the Cartesian doubt, is where the foundation of truth lies for me in the Western World. Descartes writes in *Meditations* I, that when he is sitting by the fire writing his essay, he comes to the assumption that he is truly doing this (Descartes P7), but how is he supposed to completely know?

I am not a fan of the Evil Demon argument that Descartes writes about in the *Meditations*, but I do appreciate it when he questions his sanity. The Evil Demon just seems like a fairy tale of some sort. I see no way to infer that there is some Evil Demon tricking my mind and experience at every turn. The problem I have come to see with all my misdeeds and behaviors was my ignorance, and the more knowledgeable I have, the better my actions have become. Ignorance and misunderstanding are the only true evils there are. Such philosophers as Pseudo-Dionysius would say, "By aspiring to the non-existent, they aspire to the evil." Ignorance is something that does not exist. Ignorance is just a lack of knowledge. That is why it is evil. When we aspire to error in thinking and come to false conclusions is where all evil is. So, I do not see a Being that is all knowing as being evil; therefore, there is no logical inference for an Evil Demon, but everybody has experienced someone who is insane.

Insanity is something everyone has an experience with if they live in a big city. Therefore, I like Descartes' argument for the question: how do I know I am not mad? Anyone who lives in San Francisco, every time they walk downtown, we all see crazy homeless people talking to themselves all the time. We all have these experiences witnessing their insanity, and I would say most of us do not give it a second thought, but something I have asked myself, just like Descartes in the *Meditations* when he is sitting by the fire, how do I know that is not me? How do I know that is not me being a crazy homeless person in San Francisco? How do I know that every conclusion that I have come to in my life is nothing but a psychotic delusion? How do I know that is not me digging through a trash can, yet I think I am a philosophy major at SFSU studying Wilfred Sellars? I truly have no way of knowing! But, if I am trapped in that state of mind, the only way I would ever be able to get out of it is to be able to doubt my circumstances. This is what Descartes does when he is sitting by the fire in the *Meditations*. Descartes is questioning his sanity. If he was insane, then he would only be able to get to the knowledge that he was through doubt, and Descartes knows this. I, myself have had my own experiences with insanity, and it was only through questioning my sanity that I was able to get out of it and function in society.

The problem with an insane person is that they are not able to ask themself the question: "Am I truly sane?," and, from what I have noticed, most "sane" people cannot ask themselves that question either, and everyone believes things that are not true in an empirical world of relativity and duality (Maya), especially in the age of information. So, one of the key questions I was able to ask myself is: what is the difference between a false belief and a delusion?

There are two main different realities in American politics with MSNBC and Fox. They cannot both be right because they are opposite concepts of political reality in every way. So, this is proof that everyone believes things that are not true in the age of information, and the people that watch these different concepts of reality believe it for no other reason than someone told them, it fits their experiences, and it makes them feel good and even reinforce what they already believe. It is also important to note that it was Reagan repealing of the *Fairness Doctrine of Reporting* that allowed for biased new sources like Fox and MSNBC to form. I would argue most people seek their news shows for the information they want to believe be it MSNBC, Fox, or CNN in the age of information, and I cannot even begin to explain the problems Facebook is causing with the realities of all Americans, let alone the world! The United States Congress is having hearings about this now to find out what to do with relative information of social media giants such as Facebook and the problems they are causing in our societies. Yet, we all seek relative information for the same reason: a validation of our individual experiences.

It is also important to acknowledge how many of the people that watch those different shows, with different forms of reality, ever ask themselves the question: Am I truly sane? I would argue not too many of us do! So, if a sane man cannot question his sanity, or even his relative reality, that he is seeking this information for no other reason than comfort of opinion, and believes things that are not true by doing this, which we all do, be him truly sane or insane, then what is the difference between a sane and an insane man if both believe things that are not true, and neither can question their sanity? I use nothing but the election of Donald J. Trump to show how completely crazy all Americans are!

It is amazing the people that support Trump back him for all kinds of concepts they hold to be true, like sexual morality, and Trump proved to them in video in the 2016 election that he was not sexually moral in anyway. Yet, they listen to people like Tucker Carlson preach these ideas and shout sex is between one man and one woman from the mountain tops! Tucker Carlson in his nightly reporting is always pointing to some sexual deviant who is a Liberal is some way, and you can see how he is trying to scare his own viewers with this information! Yet, I have seen a three-minute video on Donald J. Trump sexualize his own daughter on Howard Stern! It is a YouTube video where is says several extremely disturbing things he wants to do sexually to his own daughter! I ask his followers to watch it and they flip out! Here is the link: https://youtu.be/DsOVVqubBus . It is nothing by pride and ego to say you are all about sexual morality and marriage, or against any sexual relations that are not just between one man and one woman and then vote for a man for President of the United States who has twenty-five creditable accusations of rape, confessed to it on tape, and sexualizes his own daughter over and over to the eyes of the public! There is not one Democrat that I have talked to that is in favor of any of Trump's sexual conduct in any way!

It is not just Republicans that have too much pride in American politics as well. Being in San Francisco I am in a very Democratic city. San Franciscans love Civil Rights for all. Yet, you point out to most San Franciscans that all their Civil Rights stem from one place: a radical interpretation of *The Book of Matthew*, and they freak out! It is well known American History that Dr. Martin Luther King Jr. was a Doctor of one thing: Christian Theology. Any San Franciscan I point that out to usually gets quite offended! I've told several of them that King got it from Gandhi, and Gandhi based it on Thoreau, and that both Gandhi and Thoreau were pro-Christ anti-Christian as I argued in favor of in *Pseudo-Laws and Pseudo-Morals* and that we all just have the same two problems: ignorance and understanding which are the only true evils in this world, but it is amazing to see the overwhelming majority of all San Franciscans I have ever talked about where Dr. King got his ideas get extremely angry and offended. Nonviolent peaceful protest is all about loving your enemy, and it is nothing that is a secret in any way! They just refused to believe it! Just like people who support Trump refused to believe he sexualizes his own daughter and is guilty of rape! This is evidence to me that we all believe things that aren't true if a man like Trump can win President of the United States and Democrats refuse to acknowledge that people that they disagree with ideologically don't have "truths" in their doctrines too!

Both sides, be them Democrat or Republican, make the bombastic claim that America was founded on Freedom, when any historian can easily show how America was founded on Colonialism, and Colonialism was nothing but supremacy and genocide! Karl Marx makes some very good arguments on his book on religion that Christians were nothing but Satan worshipers using the history of Colonialism to prove his point! He said only Satan would sacrifice his only child and eat him, and he used nothing but the terror that all the Colonialists did to all minorities around the whole world to prove his point because they did it all in the name of Christ! They killed and conquered everywhere they went! It is why Thoreau was pro-Christ anti-Christian. Thoreau dealt with this type of discrimination in his day and age. Thoreau was born about forty-two years after the end of the Colonial era in 1817, so he lived much closer to that age of discrimination. The fact that most Americans still to this day say America was founded on freedom, even if they are a minority, gives proof that all of humanity believes things that aren't true for no other reasons that it fits our experiences and validates what we all already believe, which is nothing but what pride truly is. Pride is the demon that *Bible* talks about for this very reason. Pride gets us all to believe things and take them as true for no other reason that it fits our experience and makes us feel good out the reality our own minds put us in; therefore, doubt and looking is much more fundamental to knowledge than seeing is for knowledge because seeing is something that animals are stuck in.

If an animal has a hallucination of any kind, they would have no way to question it, so in the Space of Reasons looking is the Cartesian gift that humans are blessed with, and when someone says, "we can always be wrong" that is what they are truly holding the claim to whether they acknowledge it or not, and Sellars states "there is no such thing as a non-inferential belief" (Sellars P135). That, to me, means all beliefs in their essence are cases of looking in the Maya because it is only through looking that we get to what we infer, and these beliefs are structured semantically with the interaction we all have with our fellows through psychological nominalism. We can admit that we can always be wrong because it is nothing but an inference, and inferences can always be wrong, which shows some level of skepticism and Cartesian doubt. This means, that if Sellars admits it or not, looking is more fundamental to finding what is true because any belief can be wrong because it is nothing but an inference, and if one wants that correction, they need to allow for the Cartesian doubt.

Sellars not only talks about ties in *Empiricism and Philosophy of the Mind*, but Sellars picks geometric shapes to write about all the time. In *Section V Impressions and Ideas: A Logical Point*, Sellars writes about *"sensations of red triangles"* (Sellars P55). Sellars writes about Jones experiencing a red triangle, and Sellars is quick to point out that it is an experience only if it is true. He says this experiencing is in a case seeing, and with this seeing it would be an endorsement. What I want to point out to Sellars is that he has no way of knowing if it is a seeing and Sellars admits that when he states, "if its propositional content were true" (Sellars P54). So, Sellars is wanting it both ways. He is claiming he can call it a seeing if it were true, but he has no way of proving to us that it is true because it is nothing but a belief, and as Sellars wrote a belief is nothing but a semantical inference. If it is a seeing or some type of delusion, and Sellars is admitting this with that claim "if," even though he calls it a seeing. This to me shows that even Sellars admits there is no way to truly call it a seeing.

When it is triangles that Sellars is describing that Jones is seeing I also want to point out that there is no such thing as a Euclidian triangle. There are objects in this world that are triangular but is proven in the modern mathematics that triangles either have more or less than 180 degrees; therefore, there is no such thing as a Euclidean triangle. This was proven only through looking, and it is the falsification that space is Euclidean that lead us to a better understanding of the true geometry of the Maya.

Immanuel Kant made the claim that space was Euclidean, and he stated it with apodictic certainty. To me there are only two things that I can say with apodictic certain, and to be apodictic means to be incontestable through experimentation. There is no more certainty than apodictic certainty, and this is what I believe through my own inference that Kant was after: certainty! Not truth, but certainty, which is a fearful disposition to be in if one can admit it or not! To have certainty would be to be free of all fear. The only things I can take that are apodictically certain are: one: that I exist, which goes to the Cartesian foundation of truth, and two, any other conclusion I come to, besides the fact that I exist, I could be wrong about, which also goes with Cartesian doubt. So, existence and the uncertainty of this Maya are the only things that are apodictically certain. Everything else is an inference, and it is an inference based on psychological nominalism because that is how beliefs are formed, and as Sellars points out, as I stated above, all beliefs are a matter of inference. For me all I have is what I believe, and the more I claim as certain, the less answers I am able to get to because I need to always allow for the self-correcting through falsification and doubt.

In *The Philosophy of Space and Time*, by Hans Reichenbach, Reichenbach goes on to destroy Kant and his claims that space is Euclidean with apodictic certainty. Reichenbach wrote this book after Einstein and the Einsteinian Relativity which gives us a better understanding of the empirical world than when Kant was alive. It was the ability to look at space-time and take every triangle as either having more or less than 180 degrees, that enabled Reichenbach to write this award-winning essay. Reichenbach shows throughout the book that the rules of Euclid only exist in one place: The Space of Reasons. It is only in the mind where a triangle has exactly 180 degrees. It is only in the mind where two parallel lines never get farther away from each other, and they never get closer together either. Only in the mind with the construction of thoughts through empirical impressions are the rules of Euclid true, and the mind, or The Space of Reasons is only imagination as I show throughout this book! In the inferential truth of the Einsteinian Universe Euclid and Kant are destroyed!

It is also by looking that we find problems with Einstein's theories. Dark energy is something that with our current understanding violates the General Theory of Relativity. It states in *Physic World Dark Energy and Dark Matter*, that the violation of one of physics most beloved principles: the conservation of energy, could resolve the problem of our universe expanding, and it would only be by questioning and doubting the conclusions Einstein came to that we can ever get that answer. If light were retarded over billions of light years, instead of always traveling at the same speed, which is a main premises of both the Special and General Theories of Relativity, it would violate the conservation of energy, and explain the universe to look as though it is expanding but truly is not. But, according to these theories, light remains constant at 299,792,485 meters per second, and the only thing that ever changes with light is its wavelength. But, if instead light was retarded over billions of light years, then that would explain the paradox of Dark Energy. So, all of this reinforces that to question and to doubt through looking is the biggest gift that humans are blessed with in the Space of Reasons because maybe this retardation of light and the violation of the conservation of energy could explain the quantum gravity Einstein could never reconcile with the General Theory of Relativity? Which was where my mind went right off the bat. We are all wrong all the time: even Einstein!

Looking at this light is what our constellations are about. It is only by looking at this light, and the photons which arrive from the billions of light years away, that we can measure the wavelength, and we have known for a while now that the universe is expanding. That is something Einstein was able to reformulate his theories for and disregard this Cosmological Constant, but it was not until the early 90s that we discovered this Dark Energy and that the farther away a galaxy is, the faster it is receding from us. That is only shown to us by looking and inspecting what we see. What we have always been able to see is the photon, but only by looking and questioning, do we get a better understanding of a photon and where it arrives from and what might truly be happening all these billions of light years away. This all tells me that my problem with Sellars is not so much about what he is claiming, for he allows that we can always be wrong, my problem is with the semantics he uses to make his claim. He is not acknowledging the paradoxes in an empirical world of relativity and duality, just like I pointed out in *Pseudo-Laws and Pseudo-Morals* that Thomas Aquinas would not either and why we were all stuck in the Dark Ages for so long when he was trying to reconcile "love your enemy" with "eye for eye; tooth for tooth!" We cannot say seeing is more fundamental to the truth if we can always be wrong. That means that looking is essential to finding any discrepancy of the falsification and overthrowing one theory for another. For it is only by looking that we find a problem with what we see, and what we see is expressed in the psychological nominalism.

So, my main problem with Sellars is his nomenclature, for by holding onto seeing he is making the same mistake Kant made about Euclid and Euclidean space, and that is the desire for certainty. With seeing, and the claim that seeing is more fundamental to the truth, to me, it is just a desperate attempt for certainty, just like Kant and his claims of Euclidean space being apodictically certain.

Sellars shows this again by writing, "For seeing is a cognitive episode which involves the framework of thoughts, and to take it as the model is to give aid and comfort to the assimilation of impressions to thoughts, and thoughts to impressions which, as I have already pointed out, is responsible for many of the confusions of the classical account of both thoughts and impressions" (Sellars P110). It is interesting how Sellars is admitting in this statement that these impressions we get through seeing have confusion to them. That is saying that what we are seeing needs to be looked at, including the thoughts because all our thoughts are, are those impressions of the empirical world (imagination), and one of the things I admire most about Descartes is the inspection he gives us in the *Meditations* about his thoughts, and one of the premises I have found for my thinking is that the only thing I get a panoptical view of are my own thoughts. This is something I find Descartes stating in the *Meditations*, for he is constantly questioning the objects that he sees and any type of certainty they might give him, for with Descartes looking is more fundamental to knowledge; with Descartes looking is parasitic on seeing, and that is what we do when we inspect an object: we look at it. Sellars is also acknowledging that what we see is what gives us these impressions, and yet there are things wrong all the time with these thoughts. They need to be looked at just like Descartes claims we can.

Even Sellars himself, when he came up with this ground-breaking anti-foundationalist theory, it was a case of looking. He had to inspect the empirical objects and question them. Sellars was questioning the fact that nonconceptual content could have a rational role in the mind.

As I stated my main problem with Sellars was with his nomenclature, so if I could rename one of his ideas, I would not call the mind the Space of Reason, but I would call the mind the Space of Imagination. For that to me is all the mind truly is: imagination. This is also one of the main premises of Vedanta that has led to my sanity, and that is where Euclidian geometry is as well, for Euclidian geometry only exists in one place: the mind; therefore, it is imagination. It is only in the mind, like I stated before that a triangle has exactly180 degrees as Reichenbach proves, and the mind is nothing but the amalgamation of limited impression of the empirical world and our interpretation of it which is expressed through semantics: psychological nominalism. Sellars writes about seeing red triangles all throughout his book, but those are just meant to resemble one thing that only exists in the Space of Imagination: the Euclidian triangle.

I would not call it the Space of Reasons because that Space can be both reasonable and unreasonable. Everybody's mind is both rational and irrational. People come to conclusions that are false all the time. Most Americans do as I stated above, and everyone has believed something that is untrue about something they claim to see at one time in their life. That is why that space can be irrational as well as rational. That is why that space should be the Space of Imagination. Dr. David Landy at SFSU wrote a paper summarizing David Hume, and one of the takeaways from the paper *Recent Scholarship on Hume's Theory of Mental Representations*, Dr. Landy, was that all imagination is based in empirical experience. Here Landy is using abstract ideas, just like Euclidean geometry, but he does it with the city of New Jerusalem (Landy P5). This city is nothing that has ever existed, just like a Euclidean triangle, but we can still piece it together with our mind, and we piece it together with our mind through psychological nominalism and the amalgamation of concepts that we get impressions of in other circumstances.

New Jerusalem exists in the mind and on the paper, nowhere else. Yet it was pieced together by the mind and the concept of other cities. There are all kinds of things that exist in Sellars' Space of Reasons that do not exist in reality, and there was a time that humans thought that things, such as Euclidean geometry did exist in reality, yet that has been destroyed by Minkowski, Einstein, and Reichenbach, and it is only through the power that humans have through looking that it was overcome; therefore, all but two things need to be questioned: existence and uncertainty. For it is only by questioning and doubting that we get to any type of better understanding of the truth through inference of this Maya.

Another reason that space is the Space of Imagination is that the human brain processes about 400 billion bits of information a second, but as humans we only have the capacity to comprehend two-thousands of those bits every second according to Wise Geek, a medical journal. That means that as humans we only comprehend far less than 1% of what is around us visually. That means somewhere around 99% of the empirical world is filtered out of our daily concepts and understanding of reality. Therefore, we conceived that space was Euclidean because our minds filter out most of reality. We also would not even be able to function if it did not filter all that out. Our senses would overload our minds and we would be unable to do anything. That is what drugs like LSD and other hallucinogens do. They remove the filters in between our senses and our mind. That is what people meant in the 60s when they said they were going to trip and experience reality, but it is not reality because our brains and minds have no way to process and comprehend the Maya, so we see all kinds of crazy things that are not there. It was only through looking that we were able to understand that as humans, in our everyday experience, when we are sane and sober, we are all still far from processing the empirical reality that is around us, so how could the mind be anything but imagination if we are comprehending less than 1% of reality?

I am not arguing for Pyrrho. I do not believe that I will be walking somewhere and end up stepping off a cliff. There is a pragmatism to my skepticism, just like Sellars. If I see a cup on the table, I take it as true, but if it is a hallucination, I would like to know, and if I cannot question what is in front of my mind I will never know if I am wrong. It starts with a cup on the table for me, but it could truly be anything in the Maya that I could be mistaken about.

I am also not making a solipsistic argument. I see how humanity depends upon the existence of each other. We survive together and are born in families, tribes and have developed into the modern-day society being able to achieve all kinds of things. I have no problem inferring the existence of my fellow human for the scientific documented reasons of our survival, but I am willing to question my sanity.

This question of one's sanity was the gift that John Nash was blessed with. He was one of the few people that developed paranoid schizophrenia and was able to overcome it. He did this all by questioning his sanity and the conclusions he came to. It is well documented in the book *A Beautiful Mind*, and even throughout all his insanity he still came to a rational conclusion. That is how he came up with Game Theory, which he won the Nobel Prize for. Which is amazing to show that even irrationality can lead to things that are rational because, as was stated above, all imagination is based on impressions of empirical fact. It was John Nash's hallucinations which led to all his award-winning theories. Nash would listen to the same voices that were the cause of his delusions and then would come up with all his prize-winning theories. This shows me that I will never know if I am irrational unless I can doubt my mind and the conclusions I come to. Unless we can all question what we see, and instead of seeing something as fundamental, look at it and question it for a better answer. Every book that I see and pick up looks to be a Euclidean rectangle. But that is not the case, and it is only through looking and inspection that that is revealed.

I accept the premise on faith that the empirical world exists in some form. I find the empirical world to be true only because my mind develops, and I only get better answers by interacting with the empirical world. My foundation that this world is not solipsistic is because of psychological nominalism, and the constant interactions with others that that requires. The imagination of my mind is based on the "truths" of the Maya. I also see no need for any language if this world is solipsistic. For language is for communicating from one mind to another. Dr. Mohammad Azadpur writes about psychological nominalism quite well in his essay *Knowing the Unknown*. In this essay Azadpur writes, "Such conformism produces patterns of cultural propriety (normativity), which legitimate the proper use of linguistic expressions. The intentionality of mental states is, in turn, inherited from the normativity of overt linguistic utterances via the introduction of semantic discourse." (Azadpur P39). Azadpur goes on to explicate how through semantical discourse we can articulate the truth. Azadpur writes how we can express knowledge through language, which is the psychological nominalism. It is these statements here which lead to some type of credence of my beliefs in my thoughts, and the truth of my thoughts. There would be no need for discourse if my reality were solipsistic. But it is only that fact that, as a human, I can look and come up with my semantical reality. Epistemology is only one thing for me:

the attempt to express reality through language, and it is language and the constant development we get through the interactions of others that psychological nominalism is based on as well.

As humans we have the power to look, and that is because as humans we have the power of language, and the ability to attempt to describe reality through semantics. This goes to my equation of the Mind: $((T>B)>F)>A$: thoughts rise, which lead to brain states, then feelings, and it is how we feel about what we think that controls our actions. I have struggled with psychosis just like John Nash did. I was not a full-blown paranoid schizophrenic, but my brother had the worst case of paranoid schizophrenia I have ever seen. I have been diagnosed with schizoaffective bipolar type disorder, and today because of both of my equations, the other being $((\sim T>\sim B)>\sim F)>\sim A$, which I neglect all my thinking and empty my mind daily I am basically off all my psychiatric medications. I just take 1/8 of a 5mg tablet of Saphris for sleep and CBD for my epilepsy.

I am rewriting this book because what I predicted came true with my mental exercises, which is a daily meditation of forty-five minutes laid out in my chapter on ADHD. That single pointed concentration (Trataka) is the key to each one of my chapters because it has allowed me to constantly inspect my own mind in a panoramic view, and nothing has helped me more with my psychosis and sanity then being able to inspect my mind, question my reality, admit when I am wrong, then negate every thought, even hallucinations, that rise when I see they are not true. The Negation of the thoughts, or $\sim T$, is what completely saved me recently with a medication they put me on for my epilepsy called Primidone.

Primidone is a barbiturate that metabolizes into Phenobarbital, and it works great for stopping my seizures. There was just a large problem that had arisen. The Primidone was very intoxicating and made me have hallucinations and paranoia. I also don't like feeling high anymore now that I am sober and meditate daily because I am always aware of what I am thinking and if I am not thinking clearly. I was not completely psychotic because I could tell what I was seeing was not true. That is why they were more illusions, but I did end up in the ER paranoid as well.

Like I stated I have an organic brain disorder, and with the constant seizures I have the chemicals in my brain fluctuate, which causes all kinds of psychological issues, but what I have learned how to do through single pointed concentration meditation (Trataka), is to control the brain states, or **B**, through the focusing of the Thoughts: **T**, and this allows me to either accept a feeling: **F** or go back and negate the thought: **~T**, which then allows me to have some type of control of my actions: **A**. It has been amazing and has gotten me off basically all psych-medications. I am not even having illusions at the moment, and I only take 1/8 of a Saphris for sleep. The Average does is at least a 5mg tablet twice daily which I was on for years.

I love being off these medications because just like John Nash, and just like my brother, my thoughts are completely retarded when I am on them. I have no ability to think! I could not pass a basic algebra course at City College of San Francisco while being on Clozaril. Clozaril also has more side effects than any other drug, and they rarely use it because of that, but I have been on almost every psych medication there is in the PDR at one time because I have an organic brain disorder that does not respond well to medication. I have been told by lots of doctors Clozaril is very effective, and they use its chemical structure to constantly come up with new drugs that do not have as many side effects, but I was only able to get off my psych medications by working on controlling my mind every morning for 45 minutes with Trataka as I laid out in the chapter on ADHD.

I had been off all medications for a while except the liquid CBD, and I had still been having some seizures. That is why they put me on the Primidone. I had been on Phenobarbital before, and it worked quite well. I would also say I am getting older and more sensitive to medication, so when they put me on the Primidone, it stopped my seizures completely, which only one other medication has done that for me: Lamictal. But on the Primidone, I started having illusions as I stated. I went to the emergency because my mood and psychosis was going crazy, and I could look at it and acknowledge it. I quit the Primidone because I could not function on it in society, but the doctors wanted to keep me on Primidone and just add another antipsychotic medication I had been on before called Zyprexa. I said hell no!!

Zyprexa made me gain at least 100 pounds when I was in my 20s. I am 43 now, so I am sure I would gain even more, and my thoughts would be retarded and impaired again. I am still dealing with simple partial and partial complex seizures which are not too bad being on the CBD, but I am finding today that the reason I was able to get my sanity back after being on the Primidone was the same reason I was able to get off the Saphris and all my other antipsychotic medications. I spend 45 minutes every morning controlling my brain states through my thinking. I neglect all thoughts every morning, or ~T, and just empty my mind to experience what I truly am: Consciousness. Nothing has helped my mind or sanity more than being able to question myself and exercise my mind daily. When I was coming off the Primidone, I spent a whole night neglecting every thought that came into my mind: ~T, and it completely stabilized me. I was in a hyper state of awareness and focus for a couple of days, which getting back to that hyper aware state is my constant goal. It was amazing, and it completely stabilized me, so I did not have to get on a whole bunch of medication! This is neuroplasticity. That the empirical world (Maya) is constantly shifting and our minds are meant to adapt to that shift. If we can see how our minds function, we can exercise them daily and increase all areas of our "IQ."

What I need to do, and what we all need to do, is to constantly admit when we are wrong because in this Maya it is about falsification, and falsification is all about replacing one theory for another: inference. We get closer and closer to the truth, but that is all we do if the truth is about the Maya. We continue to approach an empirical reality without ever truly getting there as long as it is too a world of relativity and duality that we are looking at. It is also through Cartesian doubt that I hold this claim of looking to be true. The only thing an animal can do is see, but as humans we have the power to look, and when we look, we can find better ways to describe our reality through semantics, and I have found I do this by the foundation of two things: existence and uncertainty. Those are the only two things I can see with apodictic certainty, and just like how Descartes creates his world with "I think; therefore, I am" so do I. Everything else in my life is a matter of looking because, as Descartes believes, looking is parasitic on seeing, and I would argue that all human realities need a parasite. We are all wrong all the time, and it is nothing but pride which causes all our conflicts as I proved in my chapter on the Law of Love.

It is only by looking that we get to overthrow one theory for another. It is only by looking that I take a book as having either more or less degrees than a Euclidean rectangle. It is only by looking, and the expression of what I find through semantics that I can approach, through inference, what truly might be, and it is a gift to be able to question my insanity just like John Nash. My delusions were not as severe as John Nash's or my brothers, but I have been able to stop the illusions and control the mood swings through the daily negation of my thoughts: ~T. This confirms my theory about the neuroplasticity of the human brain. I truly believe I have opened up new pathways through controlling the brain states through a constant redirecting of my thinking. I have been completely psychotic before talking to demons and asking them for their magic powers. I was hospitalized for it and was cutting on myself that night, and I ended up that way when a doctor asked me "now that you are sober for a year would you like to get of your antipsychotic medication Geodon?" Today I am off most medications. All mood stabilizers and antipsychotic medications are well known for retarding our thinking and limiting our functioning. That is the problem with a bipolar or schizophrenic mind. They are over producing chemicals. These medications they use to treat us makes everyone extremely stupid who tried them, are extremely expensive, and have copious other side effects.

There are two types of schizoaffective disorders. There is schizoaffective-bipolar and schizoaffective-depressive. The bipolar type is when you have mood swings which are separate from the hallucinations, which

I have been known to have. I can be psychotic without mania. If you are bipolar with psychosis, then your delusions, or hallucinations, are directly related to your mania or depression. I have been known to have had hallucinations, and illusions, separate from mood swings. This is why I was diagnosed with the schizoaffective-bipolar type because I have heard and seen things that were not related to mood swings, but I have been able to control both my moods and my hallucination through my two equations: $((T>B)>F)A$, and $((\sim T>\sim B)>\sim F)\sim A$, but as I have stated most sane people cannot question their sanity either and everyone believes things that are not true.

Pride is the greatest of all sins because pride tells us we are right when none of us truly know. We take what appears to be true as true, and as my hero Nisargadatta Maharaj states: "to take appearance as reality is a grievous sin and the cause of all calamities. You are the All-Pervading and Enteral Infinite Awareness Consciousness. Everything else is local and temporary. Don't forget what you are. In the meantime, work your hearts content – work and knowledge should go hand in hand." It is that Awareness Consciousness I try to drop my mind completely and experience every morning, as I was able to get into when I neglected every thought coming down off the Primidone. I have gotten there a couple of times, and as I stated it is slow and my mind jumps in quantum leaps. It is a very slow process and definitely not one of immediate gratification. Just realize we all fight and assume we are right instead of questioning ourselves and our sanity, which questions all my conclusions has been the key to overcoming my psychosis as it was the key to John Nash overcoming his. Sure, not everyone has struggled with the psychosis like I have or John Nash has, but none of us know if we are truly sane, and we all believe things that are not true which leads to all the conflicts in humanity; therefore, existence and uncertainty are the only two things which are apodictic in the empirical reality (Maya) of falsification in the Space of Imagination because how do any of us know we are not mad?

CHAPTER 9

Can Meditation Make a Difference for Epilepsy?

IN THE CHAPTER *The Power of Inaction* I state my equation for what controls human behavior: **((T>B)>F)>A**. Or, I put a focus on my thoughts to direct my brain states. All of that brings about an awareness and control over my feelings, which those better feelings is what brings about better actions in my life. These better actions lead me to a more purposeful and happy life without, or even just limiting, the medications I have to take. This whole book has been about everyone being consciously aware of all of our thinking so anyone who practices jnana yoga can live a more positive life. I've noticed all this only by combing silent meditation with the neurological testing I had done at UCSF. I am living a positive happy life today and am off most of the medications different doctors had me on. I am someone who had been on most of the psychiatric and anticonvulsants in the PDR at one time when I was on SSDI for over ten years. Today I am fully employed and living a productive life in society. Most people are never able to get off of SSDI, and it is a very difficult way to live because it is a very limited income. Government assistance is not a life of luxury dispute what any politician might tell someone in America.

I point out that we are all powerless over the thoughts that rise in all our minds, how we feel about those thoughts, and whether we take them as important or not. If we are truly supposed to have free will, we would all be in control of both the thoughts that rise in our minds and how we feel about those thoughts. This is because it is what we feel about what we think that controls our actions as I pointed out in *The Power of Inaction*. So, how are we any of us supposed to have any free will in any way if none of us have control over the thoughts that rise in our minds and how we feel about them? Especially if most of us are not even paying attention to 90% of what we think as both Sigmund Freud has written and anyone can find in Vedic scriptures? Also, why would anyone take any action besides what they think best suits them in the moment? The problem is ignorance and understanding for all of us as I pointed out in *Pseudo-Laws and Pseudo-Morals*. We all have with problems with our behavior because we all have problems being aware of all the thoughts that rise in our minds and how we feel about those thoughts. If there is a power of choice it is the ability to take any thought that rises in our minds as important or not, despite how a specific thought might make us feel, because it is what rises in all our minds that we are powerless over. Being powerless over one's thinking is an experiment anyone can prove to themselves. Just sit in silent meditation and try and drop your mind completely and not let one single thought rise! I infer that no beginner can!

This neglecting our thinking and the complete emptying of our minds is what lead me to my other equation: $((\sim T > \sim B) > \sim F) > \sim A$, or neglecting any thought I have that causes me or other issues. This theory has led to an amazing difference in my life, and I even had a Vedantin describe this equation as Para vairagya: Supreme Detachment. He was telling me if I practiced this perfectly, then I'd be the one in "control."

In the chapter *Awareness is the Greatest Virtue*, I showed a way of completely overcoming my ADHD without medication. I completely overcame my ADHD through meditation and focusing my mind on one thought for forty-five minutes every day. I just try to keep the words "I am" in my head every day for forty-five minutes, then I try and drop the "I am" completely too and just let my consciousness rise because all we are in our true nature is just that Perfect Consciousness. An Infinite

Emptiness. If one can experience their true Self, which is nothing but that Consciousness, or Atman, they will experience the perfection that they truly are. That is the main premise of Vedanta, which is a religion that is provable through direct experience. I am not in a continuous state of Sat-Chit-Ananda, or Being-Consciousness-Bliss, but I have had states of hyperawareness and my life continues to improve. People tell me all the time how much I have improved in my life. People are willing to talk to me who used to refuse too. I have also found all the Vedic scriptures I have explored, from all the different forms of Hinduism, go extremely well with modern science too. I have gotten rewarded over and over just by exploring Vedic concepts and ideas.

I also do believe that anyone can overcome their ADHD, as well as their anxiety, this way and they do not need to be on those specific types of medications because of the neuroplasticity of the human brain and how no one is born with an "IQ." By "IQ" I am talking all types of cognition: both social and intellectual. The mind and brain are identical to me, and the brain is meant to constantly change with our environment, which is what Neuroplasticity is all about. Both in the *Theory of Evolution* and the *Law of Karma*, which I have basically found in the *Chandogya Upanishad*, tells me this world is constantly changing and all life will either learn or it will suffer. I have found all these premises to be truly by meditating daily and exploring modern science and Vedic scriptures. I just sit in silence every day for forty-five minutes focusing on the only thing any of us can truly prove: existence. "I am" is the only thought that any of us can know with certainty. I strongly point out that this is the best way of overcoming ADHD, and it is a daily mental exercise that is not about immediate gratification. It is a slow patient practice that leads to gradual improvement, and my state of awareness continues to grow in these jumps, or quantum leaps, and so does all my cognitive function.

In *The Power of Inaction*, I point out that the neurological testing I had done at UCSF revealed to me that I had eight different brain states that my brain was constantly jumping in and out of. I am also wondering if I might have more than just eight brain states at different times because it seems as though at different times my mind is much more active than at others, and sometimes I comprehend writing or do mental exercises much easier than other times. I have also noticed the moods of my cycles, and such things as hypomania, that I have been able overcome by just scrubbing my mind free of every thought I have for only forty-five minutes each morning. It is a daily practice I never miss. I am speculating that my organic brain disorder is the cause of my ADHD as well, and that my ADHD is an organic brain disorder based on the congenital defects in my brain which cause all the executive dysfunction and other brain states and disorders. What doctors are realizing more and more now is that ADHD is just a mild form of Autism as well. I have also been able to overcome a lot of my social abnormalities through this gaining of awareness based on my daily meditation, but I still have quite a complex brain that has congenital defects they can see on an MRI.

I have what is called a Heterotopic Grey Matter. A Heterotopic Grey Matter is a nerve everyone has had from early womb to early childhood development, and it migrates from the inner part of the brain to the outer part of the brain. Bits of mine were left over adjacent to the right lateral ventricle and in the right frontal horn of my brain. This is what sends the electrical impulses. All a seizure is, is a sugar of electricity in the brain. All our brains function off of electricity, and in fact all we are is electromagnetic energy, but a seizure is nothing more than just a surge of electricity in the brain. These surges of electricity, especially over time, can cause lots of brain dysfunction, which was in the previous chapters. The Heterotopic Grey Matter is also what boosts the dopamine in my brain as well. Dopamine is the main chemical we all have in our brain for thinking; so, if I truly have any diagnosis, I will say, I have a mild form of autism with epilepsy. It is just that the Heterotopic Grey Matter sends the electrical impulses throughout my brain to cause the other disorders, even such as psychosis and mania. The structural abnormalities is what give me an organic brain disorder.

One of the things I am hypothesizing is because I have had so many seizures in my life, it is the constant seizures that have brought on the different brain states that my mind is constantly experiencing because every time I have a seizure the chemicals in my brain fluctuate. Anytime anyone has a seizure the chemicals in their brain fluctuate. I am someone who used to have constant simple partial seizures throughout the day. A simple partial seizure is a seizure that someone has where they do not lose their consciousness in, but it still sends the surge of dopamine and other chemicals throughout their brain. There would be some days I would have 30 or 40 simple partial seizures in 15 minutes, and I would get quite hypomanic, if not severally manic, because it would send the dopamine in my brain through the roof.

This organic brain disorder of a Heterotopic Grey Matter is why I have the aspects of eight different brain disorders without fitting any stereotype. The one of the things I was able to see in *Awareness is the Greatest Virtue*, is I could control and overcome the ADHD through focusing my mind every day for forty-five minutes on "I Am," and just dropping my mind completely, and the main reason I am rewriting this whole book is because everything I predicted in this chapter came true.

I am also speculating, with 99.9% of all human DNA being identical, that if ancient universal concepts can work for me, then they are work for anyone. Jnana Yoga and the neuroplasticity of the brain is what has improved my ADHD, depression, anxiety, and even mania and psychosis. I have improved all my disorders by daily meditation. I am not telling anyone to stop taking their medication, or not to trust their doctor. I firmly believe in medication if it is needed, but for lots of people I have met, it does not work, and most of them did nothing for me except give me side effects. Just like John Nash, I suffered from retardation of thoughts with the dopamine blockers and mood stabilizers, and it is wonderful to be able to think clearly and not depend on pharmaceuticals that are extremely overpriced!

I have been meditating every day for the last several years this very specific way in the chapter on ADHD, and I practice the mental exercises daily in the other chapters of this book as well. The one thing I have even seen an improvement in recently is my epilepsy. Recently, without any change in medication I am hardly having any seizures whatsoever. I will point out that I do not drink or do any drugs and have been sober 15 and a half years now. I do not even drink caffeine because caffeine is something which effects my seizures more than alcohol. I have also been told by every doctor I have talk to, that caffeine, by far, is the most under rated drug there is, but any drug that is addictive to the brain can cause or magnify seizures for anyone. I would argue most people have no idea how addictive caffeine truly is because it is so acceptable. I was having nocturnal grand mal seizures before I gave up caffeine too! Nocturnal grand mal seizures are very large ones that are tonic-clonic happening while one is sleeping, so their whole body is convulsing. But since I gave up caffeine, I do not have those either.

I do have a partial complex seizure about once a month now, but it does not last too long and I recovery very, very quickly. I just a temporary loss of consciousness and it takes about 10 minutes for all my cognition to completely return. The only medication that ever stopped my seizure completely, that was not a narcotic, was Lamictal, and I can no longer be on it because of the lethal side effect I got after being on it for fifteen years. The other medication that stopped my seizures completely was Primidone, but I do not like feeling high at all anymore. I also have no ability to function normally in anyway being intoxicated like Primidone would do to me, so I do not take Primidone. I would not be able to live a happy and productive life while intoxicated. This is why I meditate daily and just use CBD, which I do not get any intoxicating feelings from. For some people CBD can be psychoactive, but for me, and lots of other people I have met, it is not. I also take 1/8 of a 5mg table of Saphris for sleep because Saphris, which is an antipsychotic medication. I just cannot sleep without it, but I think clearly today, and if it is something I am addicted to now it is thinking clearly. I do not like feeling intoxicated in anyway anymore now that I meditate so much as well.

I speculate that all our brains are considered "plastic," so with this speculation I can control my brain states through the focusing of my thoughts daily on just the only thing any of us can take for certain:

"I Am." I have seen how this daily effort has been able to make a difference with my epilepsy too. I have been on every antipsychotic medication there is too. I have even been on Clozaril. Clozaril is a treatment for schizophrenia, schizoaffective and bipolar disorders that they only use once there is nothing else left to try because of all the side effects it has. Some people are never able to get off Clozaril either because they go even crazier without it than they did before they were on it! It seemed as though I got that side effect too, but because of the single pointed concentration meditation (Trataka) I slowly weaved myself off all of all psych-medications. I am just taking 1/8 of a 5mg Saphris for sleep. That antipsychotic medication is the only medication which has ever been able to get me to sleep. But the standard minimum dose of Saphris is 5mg twice daily. My daily dose is 1/16 of the minimum dose. Saphris is a D2 dopamine receptor cite blocker. So, it is my D2 dopamine receptors that are over producing the dopamine. Not either the D1 or D3s.

I am grateful I am not on Clozaril today because all the side effect it gave me, and just to be on Clozaril someone has to have a blood test one a week for six months, then once every other week for another three months, then once a month for the rest of your life! That is completely obnoxious! But I have been able to stabilize my mind, and improve all areas of my life, by focusing on controlling my brain states through my thinking! One of the things Clozaril did, that a lot of dopamine blockers do for me is helped my seizures, which is an atypical reaction.

Every dopamine blocker has a seizure rate. That means it causes seizures in people, not just me, but anyone. My reactions to those medications are abnormal as well. Like when I was on Zyprexa, which has the highest seizure rates of any antipsychotic. Zyprexa has a .475% chance of giving anyone a seizure, but Zyprexa helped my seizures too. This is why I also speculated at my ADHD is due to an over production of dopamine. My ADHD is more of a hypomania at least in some neurotransmitters, but I would also argue that parts of my brain are quite underdeveloped, which is what autism is. Autism is considered a social developmental disorder, or social retardation of thinking. I clearly show this behavioral issue. This also perfectly explains my complete lack of impulse control. I have not always known what is and is not appropriate to say. That, in itself, is every developmental, which is a nice word for retarded, which is the autism in me.

Today I am only on one medication for epilepsy, which is CBD! CBD comes from the marijuana plant, and it is amazing the amount of neuroreceptors in the brain that respond to the different chemicals in a positive way with the compounds in the marijuana plant. There is CBD, CBG, THC, which is the main compound this psychoactive for someone, which means gets them high, and THCV, and it is amazing that I do not have to see a doctor for any of these. I would argue that the CBD has some neurological influences on my ADHD and mood too, but the main aspect of overcoming my mood, and increasing my attention span, as well as the continuing of development of my brain, is through my daily exercises in this book.

I first started to do all these these mental exercises constantly while I was on the Saphris, then I split a nightly 5mg tablet in half and took that for six months, then I took ¼ for another six months or so, then for about another three months I only took 1/8 of a 5mg tablet which is .625mg. I went a while functioning quite well with no antipsychotic medication at all. A couple of years, but I noticed I just wasn't sleeping that well without any Saphris, so that I why I take 1/16 of the lowest dose. I still see my doctors, including Paul Garcia at UCSF, but it is wonderful being off all those medications. The only side effects I get from CBD is it seems to be excreted out of my pores and I smell it in the morning before I take a shower, but not throughout the day. It also seems to make my complexion a bit redder, but not a big deal considering it won't kill me like some of the others, and even my liver tests are good.

I feel like I am having less brain states because my mind is so much more tranquil now. I am developing impulse control, which happens daily with my practice. I am really not having too many seizures these days either. I can read and pay attention to anything, so my ADHD isn't an issue. My hypomania has subsided, and I can get to that state of complete emptiness at times, but as I stated it is not about immediate gratification. It is a slow patient improvement that is a daily practice that everyone, no matter who they are, if they struggle with mental illness or not, will find impossible when they begin to drop their minds completely and just get into their true Self: Consciousness. The type of meditation I do is a daily mental exercise that I have found completely rewarding in every way.

So, if you are looking to make a difference in the way you live your life, or the way you look at the world. If you are wanting to be able to happy no matter what is going on in the world, then do not just settle with medicine. Try the Eastern approach to life and combine it with western medicine because Vedanta is extremely compatible with Western Science. Vedanta is just like science. It uses no blind faith! None! The Rgveda is the one ancient document that nothing in modern science has disproven. Just realize that the mind is nothing but imagination, and realize thoughts only have power over your brain states and emotions if you take them as true instead of as just imagination. Those are the concepts of Vedanta: the mind is nothing but imagination, and that Ananda, or bliss, is within you, and what you are at your core at is nothing but Consciousness. I have gotten in touch with that Ananda by clearing out all the thoughts, or vasanas, from my mind a couple of times, so I have experienced it at time. I am just working on being in that state of mind every minute of every day now.

I was talking to a gentleman I am friends with who is a high functioning autistic of the classic form. Anyone can tell just by talking to him he is autistic. So many more people are getting diagnosed with autism now because lots of doctors and seeing that ADD and ADHD are just middle forms. I was unable to get an appointment at UCSF with last year with the autism department because so many people are being diagnosed with it now. They have lots of the same symptoms. Autism is just much more severe form of ADHD is what some new theories are, but this gentleman I was talking to with a severe form of Autism was unable to smile because of his brain did not have the capacity to. I have seen this man laugh at certain times, so I do not believe that is completely true, but I was encouraging him to look in the mirror and think happy thoughts to and try to practice smiling daily. He did not seem to understand why I was saying this, and I was not able to explain it to him in a way that would get him to practice it daily, but my hope was for him to practice developing his brain like I have with mine with these Eastern based practices. I have my hopes for anyone that they can improve their cognition through awareness and daily exercises of the mind. For anyone to change for the better they need awareness, and that is why I recommend single pointed concentration meditation (Trataka) to anyone! Anyone at all!

I have gotten more and more awareness since I have been meditating every day in the exact way as specified by Nisargadatta Maharaj and in the Bhagavad Gita. Just focus on all any of us truly know is certain: "I am," then gently drop your whole mind and get into just your Consciousness because awareness is by far the greatest virtue of any human, and the true Self is nothing but this Consciousness controlling the universe that anyone can experience. The issue is we all think we are right about the empirical conclusions we all come to throughout our day. We all can only be certain of one think: existence! We all just have what we believe, and when we realize what we believe is nothing but imagination, with all the conclusions we all come to, that is when we have the power to shape and improve your brain states and our realities. Vedanta and Western Science go hand in hand, and this book is about what Vedanta has done for me! It has made a difference in every area of my life! So, I'm speculating Vedanta can with anyone else too!

CHAPTER 10

Digital Dementia, Brain Damage, Rebuilding Memory, and Developing Cognition

I AM SOMEONE WHO LIKES impress people with my memory constantly. It is an egotistical thing I have done throughout my life. The point of Vedanta is we are neither our bodies nor our minds. So, my mind, or anything to do with it, is not who I truly am. Both the body and my mind would be the ego in Vedanta, which the ego needs to let go of completely if we are going to discover "reality." The True Self, or Atman, in me is the True Self in you in Vedanta, which is nothing but the Pure Consciousness that is the Brahman (God). But, to tell anyone the truth, I had to rebuild my savant skills of my memory completely when I got sober because of the seizures I had from my epilepsy. The drugs I abused also made those seizures worse, and it was those seizures with the drug usage that gave me some brain damage.

Nothing enhanced the brain damage to my memory, and other cognition, like the drug speed. Nothing is worse for either the brain or the body that speed, especially if you are an epileptic. I had to work very hard on my memory daily, just by exercising it and quizzing myself on stuff I was trying to memorize. It was only the daily mental exercises that brought my memory back and have even enhanced my memory with pictures and other things like remembering names.

Remembering names was something I was always quite terrible at because I am someone who does not think in pictures in anyway. Only thinking in words is something that is abnormal. Most people think in pictures and words, then there are those who only thinking in pictures, and the smallest percentage of humans only think in words.

I listened to a Buddhist monk, who specialized in meditation and helping people overcome drug addiction, tell a room full of people once that he learned from a scientific journal that the average mind has anywhere from 16,000 to 60,000 thoughts a day, and most of those thoughts are just repetitious thoughts from the previous days of their lives. The whole point of this book is to work on emptying our minds, realize that our body or our minds is not who we truly are, and acknowledge that if we all want to change our insanity, it all starts with awareness through daily meditation. Most of what we all do is nothing but the same thing over and over and we all have the insanity of expecting something different. It is why the whole world related to that Einsteinian quote. We all do the same thing over and over, and we all expect something different from it eventually because what worked once no longer does. It is not until we respond to our pain and consequences that we can change to a better life. The Buddhist Monk also said some minds have other 60,000 thoughts a day, and he agreed when I shared that mind my sure did because he knew me for over 20 years.

The neurological testing I had done at UCSF, by Brandon E. Kopald, Psy.D., taught me serval amazing things about my memory as well. When it came to seeing the obstructed neuropathways of my brain, it was the female doctorial assistant, who was giving me the neurological examination, showed me this clue. She asked to recall certain things she had told me about earlier just a bit earlier. When she asked me, my mind then would go blank! She would then give me a little hint of some kind, and everything that I could not remember I would suddenly recall! This was also shown to me when I first started to read at Linda Mood Bell. They would ask me to describe to them what I had just read out loud and my mind would go blank, they would give me a little hint and I could recall the article, or I would reread it, and everything I was reading would come right back to me with the feeling of familiarity. I could tell I had read it all before!

This recollection told me that these memories were registered somewhere in my brain because I could recall what I had just read with a little hit. It was as though there was this obstruction in the neuropathways from the brain damage, as well as my brain jumping in and out of those eight different brain states, because of my history of all the seizures I constantly had from the heterotopic grey matter. All these issues, as well as my dyslexia, ADHD, and autism, I believe, obstructed my ability to recall things that had just been told me, or I had read, even five minutes before.

Something which also made it quite difficult for me to even try and recall anything was to be able to pause in any way because, as was stated, my neurological impulse control was at a frightening zero! I say frightening because that doctorial assistant seemed terrified and gasped when she told me: "you have exactly zero impulse control!" This lack of impulse control has been one of my biggest problem my whole life.

Nothing, absolutely nothing, has helped me more than the ability to pause, which I have only gotten through meditation. That ability to pause has also helped me work on rebuilding my memory by opening up the pathways where those memories where stored. Just to be able to sit even 30 seconds to try and work on recollecting a specific name or get to the end or a paragraph and quiz myself on what I had just read. I still quiz myself on names when I am work. I practice on recollecting names from the customers I am looking up in the computer. In the past, I would always just give up when I was searching for a customer's name in the computer system. Now I look at their name on the report, go the computer, sit for just 30 seconds at the most, which was impossible at first, and lots of times I can recall the specific name. The more I try on memorizing different things, the easier it gets. So much of what we do is just training our minds (brains) to adapt to this shifting world around us (Maya), and all of this comes with awareness.

One of the main things that makes be believe we are not born with "IQ's," for lack of a better term, is how I have been able to rebuild my memory after all these issues. By "IQ" I am always talking social, emotional, and intellectual. Not just this 0-180 scale, but a generic term for all kinds of intelligence. Given all that, I exercise my mind daily rebuilding my memory closer to that numerical recollection I had earlier in my life and have even expanding upon it. That memory I had is known as a rote memory. I am now extremely good at quoting literature verbatim, which some Doctors in philosophy find quite obnoxious and threatening, but what is truly amazing, and gave me the idea of training my mind to overcome mental illness through jnana yoga, was I was a functional illiterate for most of my life. The Linda Mood Bell program that I took is about developing parts of the brain that are underdeveloped with people who have learning disabilities, by increasing the oxygen flow to them through daily intense exercises. In each of my chapters it is about daily exercises to developing my brain by increase all areas of intelligence that it possibly can. This empirical world is constantly shifting, and all our minds are meant to adapt to that shift. Nobody is born with an "IQ."

That ability to develop the parts of my brain that were underdeveloped at the Linda Mood Bell program is what really convinced me to rewrite this book. I had always wanted to be a writer as a child, and I wrote those poems that I open up this book with as a child. I had a third-grade reading level when I wrote them in high school, and for most of my life, I could not process and comprehend anything in more than a couple of sentences at a time. If I had written anything, I always needed someone to help me with the spell checker on the computer because I could not even decipher words from each other that the spell checker would give to me as a possible correction for the spelling error I had made. That is how terrible my English skills were. I am still not that great of a speller still to this day, but I can read and comprehend anything in English now, I am much better at catching my own typos, and I have no problem with the spell checker either. Linda Mood Bell also told me that spelling is the last aspect of reading to increase for anyone who is dyslexic, but my biggest problem when it came to reading was absorbing what I read and truly comprehending it. I can read such books as *The Enneads* now! *The Enneads* is an Ancient Greek literature from Plotinus, the first of the Neoplatonist. The average citizen cannot read that book, nor would they like to try, but this is why it is more about training our brains to do different things as soon as we are aware a part of our mind is not working correctly: develop our "IQ's" throughout our lives is part of the *Theory of Evolution* as well, and I as state throughout this book the *Theory of Evolution* and the *Law of Karma* tells me the same thing: the only thing that remains constant is change and I either learn or I suffer.

What I did for my numerical memory, or rote memory, when it was damaged was whenever someone gave me their new phone number, I would type it into the texting app on my iPhone instead of entering their contact information with name and number. This meant I had to recollect and quiz myself on their number in the texting app if I was going to contact them because I could not type their name in and get the number automatically. This was difficult and is something to this day I still work on. It is also something anyone at any age can do to enhance their memory. I would argue everyone can practice quizzing themselves with the info on their smartphones because I have seen homeless people with smartphones in the country now, and one of the bigger issues our society is having is the Digital Dementia brought about by this smartphone technology. Digital Dementia is all about the mental health issues with smartphones we can all experience. These "smart" phones causes such issues as retardation of thoughts and memories, adult ADHD, and depression and anxiety.

With the retardation of thoughts, when all we do is record things with our smartphone, instead of committing them to memory, we lose our capacity to remember anything when we need too. This tells us the brain is meant to be exercised daily with our interactions in the empirical world (Maya). With my grandmother, first she lost her hearing, then she lost her eyesight. Once she lost both her hearing and eyesight, her mind quickly faded. We all need to exercise our minds daily by engaging with the Maya around us no matter what our age. When we see how our own minds function, through things like neurological testing, and the observation of awareness through daily meditation, we can work on what needs to be rebuilt or enhanced in our own cognition.

When I first got sober, I would spend hours tying numbers into the search box of the smartphone's texting app. If the phone number pop up right away, I would know who the name and phone number of the person I was thinking about was in my mind. If not, I would have to hunt through a list of hundreds of numbers or so till I found it. It was a daily effort, and I messed up a lot of the time. When I would meet those people sometimes it would shock them when I could quote their phone number too them. It was funny because sometimes some of those people thought I was coming onto them when I did that, or it would just scare them because most people in this day and age don't know anyone's number besides their own. But just realize, that the average citizen of Ancient Greece would memorize the *Iliad*. The *Iliad* is a poem which is over six-hundred-pages! This tells me that there is so much of our memories we are not using these days, and this "smart" phone technology can make it better or worse!

My biggest problem with smartphone usage is how they are causing all kinds of neurological issues to everyone, like Adult ADHD. Adult ADHD is caused by all of the notifications that are constantly going off on them. With my ADHD, I have to make sure all the notifications are completely off my phone except something that is extremely important like a call or a text from someone. I cannot proceed in my daily activities without all the notifications being taken care of on my smartphone with my OCD. It is also my obsession to detail that they neurological testing at UCSF showed as well that makes my day impossible to proceed when I have a notification that is not taken care on my phone. "Smart" phones have the capacity to make us all much, much stupider and cause all kinds of problems.

Smartphones are even causing mental health issues such as depression and anxiety because people go onto Facebook constantly throughout their day and are comparing their miserable lives to what they see others' showing the world. What people post on Facebook is not reality. They are posting information for approval. When we all go onto these platforms like Facebook, we are just looking at what others what to show us about that they think is cool so they can get a like or a love mark on their post. None of us are seeing reality in anyway. We are just seeing what someone wants to show us so that person can get approval. Not what their life really is. When we go onto Facebook, we are comparing our insides to another person's fantasy, so it makes us depressed and anxious because our lives are not as good as the fiction someone else is showing us. We feel hopeless and inadequate because everyone else has these "wonderful" lives, so we think.

I pointed that out to a girl who was suffering from lots of medical issues I made friends with on Facebook. I told her, "Facebook is not reality. It is just what they want you to see of them. They want attention, which is just their addiction to everyone else's approval of them. Everyone suffers. Not just you and not just me with our physical disabilities, but everyone. Suffering is a key principle of life and one of the two ways we learn. The other is pleasure. We all experience pleasure and pain to varying degrees. Don't look to Facebook for reality." She had severe disabilities, so she always felt inadequate anyways. She was doing what we all do, especially when we are on Facebook: Comparing how she felt to how wonderful she saw others have it in their lives. Jealousy is a sin for that very reason. It messes up our minds and causes all kinds of psychological issues which we take out on others and ourselves.

The main problem with smartphones is that smartphones stimulate the same parts of the brain as drugs and alcohol, which will cause a chemical imbalance as well. When we boost pleasure centers in the brain, they get depleted, and when they go way up and way down too much, that throughs the chemicals in our brains off. This chemical imbalance happens especially with smartphone technology! I am completely against legalizing gambling on smartphone technology, which is on the ballot this November of 2022 in California, for this main reason especially! I see that causing nothing but chaos throughout a society that does not need any more addiction issues. It also consolidates wealth to people who don't need it, takes money away from Native American Tribes, and will enhance other addictions and isolation issues, which will cause even more mental illness throughout society!

I was given and IQ test in the fifth grade, most likely because they thought I was too stupid. I had gotten Fs in every grade except the 3rd, and that was only because of an amazing teacher Ms. Write. In the fifth grade I had gotten Fs all semester as well, but on that IQ test I was able to recite 12 digits backwards, which is as high as they go on the IQ test. I got a score of 124 on my IQ test as a kid, and that is in the top 5%. I was about twelve years old at the time. That immediate recollection was gone at one time because of the brain damage from the seizure and the different levels of cognition from the brain states that my brain is constantly jumping in and out of. I do have a video I made of me talking to a college philosophy class in a class I took called *The Philosophy of Personal Development*. In this video I wrote the first thirty-nine digits of Pi, the first twelve digits of the first seven irrational square roots, which is just 2 thought 10, and the first thirty-two digits of Euler's number all on the blackboard boggling all their minds! I have rebuilt that recollection dramatically! I would also argue most people can do this with daily practice! That recollection of the average citizen of Ancient Greece reciting the *Iliad* is my main argument for that.

I have been able to increase my social "IQ" skills as well, especially recently, but only with this awareness. If we are not aware of what our brain's defects are, we will never be able to address how our individual minds fall short. It always starts with awareness, and 90% of any problem is the ability to recognize it. The only way for any of us to truly see how our own minds function is daily meditation. Especially single pointed concentration meditation (Trataka) because it is so difficult, and it will show all of us what we are always thinking, where I mind is always going; therefore, what is truly controlling us. If you spend enough time doing it, you will realize your mind will always continue to go back to the same places. With Trataka, what controls you will always be shown to you for this very reason. You will be able to address the defects of your mind and behavior through this recognition and awareness.

As I have stated before, I do not think in pictures whatsoever, so any memory I have is all verbal, which was a huge problem with learning how to read in Linda Mood Bell program. It made them quite nervous when they found out because their whole system is about trying to get the student to draw a picture in their mind with the words they just read. I noticed that I did not really process symbols all that well with my dyslexia too. This is where I got myself to use my smartphone to enhance my cognition again!

It is proven that video games are a good thing to help increase anyone's IQ. There is lots of evidence that it is not just me that can do this. There are all kinds of website that are about brain games and increasing IQ, but anyone can also get a memory game on their smartphone for free. It is just matching one picture with another. I also realized it was working on my visual memory that helped me processes the word cognition and process the information on the pages as well as recollect them. My visual memory was quite terrible, so just processing what I read was probably even more difficult for me than some others who have ADHD and dyslexia. I am someone who needs to meet someone a couple of times before I could recall their face at all.

The reason I believe my brain did not learn to think in pictures at all was because I was basically blind as a kid without my parents knowing it. I had extremely terrible eyesight. I could not see much and no one even new till I was about five and my mom took me to the doctors for glasses. I put them on, the doctor pointed out a picture to me and said this is a tree, then I shouted, "Wow! A Tree?" That is when my mother started crying hysterically because she just realized I had not seen much of anything besides light my whole life. Remember 90% of what someone learns happens between the ages of one and five, so if I could not really see at all for those years of my life, my brain did not learn to develop that at the prime time of my life that it should have.

Not being able think in pictures is also an extremely good argument of why I am so good with verbal communication. It got those parts of my brain to be over developed in that time of anyone's life where they learn the most. My first words to anyone was to my mother when she handed me a strawberry when I was on her back and I said, "Thank you."

That gave her tears of joy because not too many little kids first words are "thank you." Most little kids do not have any word that really means much as their first word. It is just a random word, but the words I used was for an exact purpose, which was of gratitude, but either way, I only think in words. The majority of all people think in both pictures and words as I stated, and Einstein was someone who only thought in pictures and is why they said he had a delay in speech when he would talk to people. Einstein's delay in speech was about needing to process the pictures in verbal communication.

When I was in Portland Community College, at the age of 18, I had a 3rd grade reading level, and passed two classes with an A: Astrology and Music. I did not even read the book! I was really unable to read full pages at the time I took those classes. I was completely an auditorial learner who took amazing notes by hand, and I typed them up. I also had my little sister do the spell check for me on the computer. I would tell her what I wanted for the different words because my reading was so terrible. She would select the right word for me each time. That is how bad my reading and especially my spelling was, but those two classes I got A's! My teachers even asked me for my notes in both classes because I passed them out to the whole class, and everyone basically got A's!

People with learning disabilities are known to overcompensate and over develop parts of the brains that the average person does not in the early stages of their lives, because of the issues they have in functioning of other parts of their brain. It has been only within the last hundred years or so at the most that the average citizen of any country needs to be a good reader in order to get a job. That is one of the arguments for dyslexia and why so many people have it in the common day: human evolution. They have deficiencies with certain cognitive abilities, that are just now needing to be utilized in our societies, so they over work and over develop the parts of their brains that work quite well and are already at good functioning level of cognition. Most dyslexics are good with math. I am very good with math. That is why Einstein was so good with math. It as a part of his brain that did not have any deficiency and that parts of our brains were over developed because we struggled so much with the reading and writing. It got us to engage and enhance the parts of our brains that used math.

Einstein had to go to a special school too to read and write as a kid. His brain is held in the Mutter Museum in Philadelphia and was shown to be smaller than the average brain! Some say he was on the Autism spectrum as well, which more and more people are being diagnosed with Autism all the time these days. It is impossible to get any appointment with an Autism specialist at UCSF because so many kids are now being diagnosed with Autism. It takes years even if they allow it. That is how many people are being diagnosed with it recently. Bill Gates is a good example of another famous person on the Autism spectrum, but it has taken me years of practicing reading and writing daily to get anywhere with writing. Steven King in his book on writing can be summed up like this: read and write daily if you want to be a good writer! Just like I am saying meditate daily if you want to get over your mental health issues by increasing awareness and cognitive abilities to see where your own mind falls short, and practice committing things to memory daily if you want to increase your memory. So much of what we do is nothing but repetition.

Overcoming this brain damage is something I encourage every epileptic to do when I talk to them on social media, or even someone with a stroke. Some of them get offended when I tell them: "don't give up and practice daily," because I show them the video of me putting those numbers on the board and they don't think they can do it, nor do they want to try. They also do not want to give up using their smartphone technology for their memory because it is easy, convenient, and addictive. I have also been able to demonstrate to my neurologist, Paul Garcia, I have two-hundred-sixteen phone numbers in my head. I had him and his student quiz me on them after I rebuilt it completely! We all can increase our memories! Sure, some it will be easier for some than others, but our intelligences is just as much to do with circumstances as it does with our genetics. Nobody is born a genus! They develop it!

To demonstrate the obstructions of my pathways: One of the other things that I never used to have any type of dyslexia with was numbers. People with dyslexia never have problems with intermixing numbers. I noticed since my brain damage that I intermixed numbers as I do with letters now. Especially if there are two numbers that are identical that come together. Like with pi, 3.1415926535897 93238462643383279502884197, which are the first 39 digits, but when writing them and saying them out loud at the same time, I would have to catch myself not mixing them up when I was writing them on the blackboard to the class. This was never an issue before the brain damage. Dyslexia is not numerical, but because of my high level of executive, or neurological, dysfunction, based on the copious seizures I had, I would usually mess two numbers up that were identical with the next number that was not. Like with Pi above sometimes I would write 443 instead of 433. This shows me an issue I never had before all because of these seizures. The pathways were obstructed and damaged with the numerical aspects of my brain now as well. This is something I am aware of and am able to work daily too. I still work with numbers all the time. I do accounting for a living. I edited books for hotels daily, so I am meant to catch other people's mistakes with numbers, and I am constantly correcting my own at the same time now too. This also tells me that my brain adapted and tried to reroute parts of my brain functions with numbers that were damaged, to the dyslexic parts that were underdeveloped.

One of the most interesting things I have taken to be true is something I read in the book *Brains that Work a Bit Differently*, they stated that people with autism and ADHD are known to have extremely well rote memories. It is why I have always been so good at memorizing phone numbers and things that I hear over and over. Numbers themselves only go from 0 to 9, then they will always end up repeating themselves the more they expand, so people with good rote memories are known for the memorization of numbers like in the movie Rain Man, and that movie was inspired by a true individual.

Something it said in that book: *Brains that Work a Bit Differently*, which I have noticed recently for myself, is that if someone with an extremely good rote memory will try and expand their memory to memorizing all kinds of things, their rote memory will decline. I am noticing it is much harder for me to commit anyone's phone number to memory as easily as I have been able to in the past now that I am working on memorizing all kinds of things like people names and processing pictures. Today, I constantly try to memorize all kinds of things: pictorial and verbal.

But I want to reiterate the issue all developed societies are having with smartphones. The smartphone companies are also doing a good job at keeping lots of this new info out against them off the web too! They do not want their profits going down, nor do they want the bad press of the mental issues these devices cause, which could easily cause government regulation they do not want. Facebook as worked extremely hard to keep from any government regulation. Just like corporate executives did their best for a long time to hide all the mental issues in the NFL from the damaged brains of the football players. Smartphone technology is making lots of us much, much stupider!

It was my math tutor at Discovery Academy, Mr. Edwards, told me: "technology is the only thing that rises in exponents and decreases in value." The biggest problem with smartphones is they are being used as people's memory and even some basic brain function. The average person in America is recording things on their phone instead of trying to commit anything to memory. I would say reading comprehension is going way down too because people want to listen to books instead of reading them, but we can overcome this with fun as well like video games on these devices and finding things we enjoy reading. I also see commercials for these brain supplements that I have a big problem with like Prevagen.

A big issue with dementia in elderly patients is complacency. They are in a retirement home with nothing to do, so they do not do anything, then their minds slowly slip away from them. Complacency is a huge problem with dementia patients. I take a wild king mushroom supplement, it is just the same type of mushrooms we put in salads, not a hallucinogen, and they are known to help cognition. I am trying it out, but you see these Prevagen commercials make it seem like all you need to do it take this brain supplement and you'll have "a memory like an elephant!" as the old mad tells the viewer. I am not saying what we eat and take as pills, or vitamin supplements, does not help the brain. I am trying that wild kind mushroom supplement, but I find that quite dishonest of these companies, just like hiding current info on the issues of mental health and smartphone technology, to say just take Prevagen and your memory will be amazing!

I exercise my mind daily with my memory and my cognition. I read daily. I meditate daily. I believe I can still work on my "social IQ," so I ask people all the time to point out my behavior to me which I do not see that clearly. I make daily rational efforts on expanding all areas of my mind. I would argue if they took this supplement, and do not exercise their minds, their minds will still slip away no matter what! It is completely dishonest to advertise to an elderly person, who wants to relax, be lazy, and enjoy their retirement, that all they need to do is take a pill!

I showed my issues with drug commercials in *The Power of Inaction*. We all want to be Einstein, but not lots of us want to put in the work! Exercise your brain daily! I would tell them to just spend 10 to 20 minutes a day on a memory game on a phone, or just quiz yourself on something you read or listen too daily if you do not want your mind to vanish with dementia! Sure, some dementia is inevitable like Alzheimer's or something with a stroke or seizure, but even with those they encourage mental exercises to increase brain function. With Alzheimer's, this daily exercise can even slow the process, but even with those disorders they have mental exercises for those patients. There is documentation that people who have more than one language they can speak lowers the risk of something like Alzheimer's, so a lot of our intellect is about daily mental exercises.

I am a firm believer that anyone can increase their "IQ" at any age because I have completely recovered my memory from brain damage, I learned how to read at the age of thirty from the Linda Mood Bell program, and so far, I have written two books, gotten two college degrees, and was in the middle of seeking my third in a master's in philosophy, but have that on hold and want to switch to law.

I dropped the philosophy classes and am wanting to switch to law because I cannot argue in favor of things I don't believe in, just to get a good grade like certain philosophy professors what you to do at SFSU in graduate school. I do not think that would be an issue with law, but it is this neuroplasticity which tells me all humans can if 99.9% of all human DNA is identical. Sure, an "IQ" is about two things: genetics and circumstances. None of us have any control over the genetics we are born with, but we can make daily efforts on our circumstances through awareness, which those circumstances do affect the genetic mutation of each one of our own cells and putting effort into learning daily with things like memory, math, and other video games is a good way to do that, and just make a daily effort to increase your "IQ" continually throughout your day.

Today, I have the ability to read and comprehend things most people have no ability to like *The Enneads*. I spent days reading things and not having any idea what it was even staying, but I did not give up. I also make a daily effort to memorize new things using pictures and words daily. It is not that hard to use a smartphone to make your smarter instead of using it to make you and your brain stupider. Just make a conscious daily effort. Today I strive for perfection and am grateful for progress. It is good to have impossible goals and standers that we have for ourselves as is written in *The Enneads*: "For it is to the Gods, not to the good, that our likeness must look: to model ourselves upon good men is to produce and image of an image: we must fix our gaze above the image and attain the likeness to the Supreme Exemplar." It is good to have impossible goals. That is what this quote is telling me. Strive for perfection, strive for God, just realize we all will always fall short with the body and the mind, for that is not what we truly are. Do your best and let go. See the deficiencies you have with your brain and work on developing them daily. There is no problem with defects of your mind as long as we all continue to try, know, and accept, we all will always fall short. Try hard but do it with self-love. Make sure to accept the fact that you have your shortcomings, and always keep that understanding of yourself in the for front of your mind, and remember when it comes to anything in this empirical world be willing to say, "who cares?" A thought is only important if your mind tells you it is! Address the paradoxes of an empirical world of relativity and duality as well, and realize our minds always tell us things out of fear because fear is one of our necessary tools for survival that we all miss use. Make sure you accept yourself no matter where you are because you were created this way for a reason, so you are perfect the way you are; it is just the paradox of life that life is about learning; so, there is always room for improvement!

Two Provable
Definitions of God

THERE ARE TWO QUESTIONS THAT stand out more than any other: What answers can I get for my life, and how will those answers lead me to happiness? With the contemplation of these questions, it comes to me that all of my answers start out with the fact that: first, I should scrutinize everything that I interpret with my senses, and second, I should question each one of the conclusions that I come to in my mind.

Each one of my beliefs I take as a rational "choice," even though "choice" to me is more of a necessary illusion for each individual to live by, by placing each one of us at the center of our own universe; is why this empirical world is meant to be our Perfect Teacher. I proved determinism with free will as all our solutions throughout this book; so, one should ask themselves, if they believe in the power of choice: why would anyone take any action other than what they think best suits them in that moment? The same two problems we all have with our actions is ignorance and understanding, just like Socrates taught, but there is truth and fallacy with each conclusion I "choose" to take as a fact, except for: "I Am;" therefore, all I truly have is conjecture except for the fact that "I Exist," even when I make any inference with an absolute statement. Inferences are nothing but langue, and words, just like perception and motion, have relative meanings to us all. Especially the word "God!"

But being able to always be wrong, except of "I Am," is why I only speculate about what I interpret with my senses because we can all admit that our senses have quite often been led astray. I showed how all of the rationalistic aspects of all our minds have been led astray because all truths that are subject to any human mind are relative all throughout this book. This shows how relativity is part of all our empirical realities, either for myself or anyone else. We need to have the perfect objective ideal of striving for an absolute empirical truth, but the only thing that does is give any of us is a better understanding of our subjective, or relative, truth. To know the absolute empirical truth in this world is beyond any human mind!

I proved paradoxes in a relative and dual universe to a Dr. of Anthropology I took class from by showing him that the paradox of Western Science is every answer, just leads to more questions! It never leads to the end of answers! Just like they predicted in both Ancient Greece and Ancient India! Our first concepts of both relativity and duality come from Ancient India, which directly influenced the Ancient Greeks. Both the Ancient Greeks and Indians whole concept was that every answer just leads to more questions! Never to the end of answers! The Dr. I pointed this out too seemed angry, but he gave up on the argument when I brought in quantum physics and such things as other universes that function off of other laws which they are now contemplating!

I showed that Dr. of Anthropology a short video on Heisenberg's Uncertainty Principle in quantum physic, and I said, "if you can mathematically explain how a quantum particle behaves as wave when we look at it indirectly, and as a particle when we look at it directly, in a way that does not contradict itself, and rewrite Richard Feynman's *QED*, which is the most accurate of all quantum theories, which explains somewhere around 98.6% of all empirical interactions by: 'an electron goes from place to place, a photon goes from place to place, and an electron absorbs and admits a photon,' to 100% accuracy, then do it? It would prove Einstein right and Bohr wrong! You would be the next Einstein and would win the Nobel Prize!"

No mathematical mind has ever been able to do that, and I am not saying someone won't solve it someday. What I am saying is it seems to be that the skeptics of Ancient Greece and India were right: every answer of this empirical world just leads to more questions in a world of relativity and duality, which is the paradox of Western Science too! We never get to the end of answers! We always just seem to get more and more questions!

With relativity, it isn't just about motion and gravity like Einstein theories, but perception and understanding which the Ancient Greeks and Indians wrote about. With duality, duality is expressed in the terms that everything that exists in the empirical world has its opposite. Because there is hot, there is a cold. Because there is a bitter, there is a sweat. Because there is pleasure, there is pain, which are the two fundamental teachers of all life. At the most fundamental level, because there is matter, there is antimatter. The philosophers of Ancient Greece and Ancient India had no concept of antimatter, but the fundamentals of what they theorized about relativity and duality hold true to this day in this empirical world!

Yet, second guessing one's nature, which is what people like Socrates taught, who I used to prove my point in the *Pseudo-Laws and Pseudo-Morals* chapter, is not something that all people do that often from what I've witnessed in this day and age. Some people, in the most developed country in the history of the world, the United States, think that this planet is only 6000 years old. They believe that their God judges them on the amount of faith that they hold in their hearts. They use computers, see doctors, talk on their cellphones, and yet hold a different concept of "truth" than some of us who do the same thing. I don't hold to that opinion, but it could be me that is wrong. Someday they may reconcile every paradox and every empirical truth!

I believe in the atom. I have yet to analyze that atom with my naked eye, for that would be impossible, yet I still believe in it. When I talk on my cellphone, I have faith that the technology is working, and I can verify that when I meet that person, I was talking to in order rehash the conversation. I have done it so many times that I take each piece of communication for granted. Yet, it is when I make assumptions that I can be led astray. There is no true proof of what is in this empirical world, which I proved in my chapter on psychosis! Any single one of us could be a paranoid schizophrenic stuck in a different reality digging through a trash can in a big city! The only thing each experience gives me which is apodictic, is the fact that "I Am!" All I have is conjecture besides the fact that "I Exist!" Every other conclusion I come to is a semantical inference all suspect to doubt, and this applies to us all in an empirical world of relativity and duality!

Being wrong is nothing that I will ever be free of when it comes to my judgements on the empirical world, and in fact, it is something I have been able to be grateful for. It has been the only way that I have been able to learn - trial and error. I am someone who has found happiness, not from getting everything that I want, but from finding answers. I have found the best answers by looking at myself and exploring why I do what I do, just like Socrates told us to do. Socrates is credited with coining the term in the West: "know thy self." Socrates told everyone that: "the unexamined life is not worth living." This is true for me. I need to be able to look at my own motivations and actions; be willing to admit when I don't know something, and look for the answers, both in myself and the world around. This is some of what we all get from the teachings of Socrates.

One of the gifts of Socrates was that he could acknowledge the truth that came across his path. Socrates got "know thy self" from a wall at a temple at Delphi, and it is through examination of what is reflected back to me, that I find my truth as well. I am an alcoholic, and the only way I have been able to find happiness is by questioning my reality. I am someone who had a bottle of Vodka by the time I was twenty every day for a year straight. I brought the weed and the alcohol to the park because I wanted friends. I would get them all drunk and high, then I would start mouthing off to everyone because I was intoxicated and could even control my mouth sober at that time, let alone drunk! This would get all the really cool and tough people to beat me up because those were the ones I loved to pick on the most! Then I would put on my headphones and hike all over town singing as loud as I could. I would usually pass out on the street and wake up strapped down to a gurney in San Francisco General Hospital three nights a week because the paramedics would drag me in. That happened for my first year I lived in San Francisco.

Sometimes I was also working that same morning. I seemed to always wake up miraculously in the ER, and just say to the nurse, "Let me go!" as I was strapped down to the gurney in four-point restraints!

The nurse would say, "Are you going to come back?"

My response was always no, but I might be back in the same hospital bed the next night because that pattern happened basically three nights a week for a whole year.

Another complication at the time was seizures. I was having seizures undiagnosed for five years, and my whole family told me I was doing it for attention. This was an experience that definitely made me question my reality. Everyone, even doctors, who didn't know what they were doing, in the middle of Provo Utah, were telling me that something wasn't happening, when in fact it was!

When I was child, the doctor they had me see at Discovery Academy gave me one EEG and told my mother I was doing it for attention because the EEG didn't show I had a seizure. Well, something I didn't know, because I was just a kid at the time, was that someone has to be having a seizure at the same time for it to show up on the EEG as an electrical disturbance in the brain. That is what a seizure is: a surge of electrical energy in the brain because that is all the brain functions off of. Electromagnetic energy is all truly are anyways! Some of our electricity is free flowing and others it isn't, but something the doctors in Provo Utah didn't seem to know is that you have to be having a seizure at the same time or it will not show up on the EEG!

I was only 15, and that idiot Doctor at Discovery Academy was the one who had an MD! He was a complete moron, and I have met lots of doctors with degrees that have no idea what they are doing! He wasn't the only one! At that school I was losing my consciousness daily at times, and those Doctors and psychologists all told me I was making it up! That happened for 5 years because of that place, and that definitely made me question reality! Yet they were the ones who did not understand anything that was truly happening, and they were the ones with the professional training!

I pointed all throughout this book that I am pro-science and the scientific method. So, no one should think that I am against medication or seeing a good doctor who knows what they are doing. Lots do, some don't! An amazing doctor, who I still see at times today: Paul Garcia, who is head of epileptology at UCSF, and who I am still in contract with about the CBD I use, was the one who saved my life and told me: "if you don't quit drinking and using you will have brain surgery or die." Every time Dr. Garcia did not have an answer for my medical condition, which was quite often he would tell me, "I don't know." That Dr. has a waiting list and is head of one of the world-renowned hospitals for epilepsy and neurology.

It was the fear of death that got me to try to get sober, but that fear did not get me to quit. It took another eight years of me trying daily, with not much success, especially with behavioral issues I had, in order to achieve any type of sobriety. I would get a couple of days, then go out and do the same thing over again. All of this led me to a quote that I heard others tell me for years. This quote was from Einstein. Einstein said: "Insanity is doing the same thing over and over and expecting a different result." To me this isn't necessarily insanity because everyone does this. That is why the whole world loved and related to that quote so much! We all do the same thing over and over all the time and expect different things to happen!

The reason why so many of are stuck in this type of "insanity" of repetitious behavior is because the only thing any of us know how to do is something which worked for us in the past, and the problem is, is if we don't know what to do, all we have is that past experience. No matter how futile and self-destructive that experience and currently be, it work at one point in our lives.

I would do this insane behavior of repetitious drinking and use of drug just hoping to get some type of relief from the conflict in my mind and soul, but it never came. The noise in my head was so loud that the only solution I could grasp onto was drinking to oblivion! It wasn't until I had the ability to look for answers, admit what "I don't know," and question myself, as well as my intentions, that I started on the road to happiness. For me, to question everything that is in my ability of perception is the only way that I have gotten any answers that have led to my happiness. I have also seen this reasoning laid in front of all of us throughout the great of history of the past! It is meant for everyone: "know thyself" and question your reality, because we are all wrong all the time!

Looking for answers is something that Socrates' student Plato writes about in the *Republic*. In the *Republic*, Plato writes how Socrates explains that God is truth, truth is good, and opinions are ignorance. Socrates then goes on to explain that the only thing that he has are his opinions. This is true for me as well because the truth for us all is relative when it comes to the empirical reality. The only thing thinking does, or the empirical impression on the brain that we rationalize, AKA mind, is prove I exist! I can always be wrong about what those impressions truly are! I will always be ignorant, and I will never fulfill the task of looking for the answers from the empirical world, so the one and only thing I can truly know is the "I."

Socrates got "Know Thyself" from the temple wall; that message has been echoed throughout history, but there was a pre-Socratic philosopher who explored his mind and soul based on his own intuition: Heraclitus. Heraclitus showed how people need to look into themselves to find peace, and that that quest will never be over.

Heraclitus was all about self-examination. To look inward is the only place that one needs to look. Heraclitus became a hermit and isolated himself from everyone so that he could explore the truth in his own thoughts. This was the only way for him to get his answers. For me, it is not about isolation, but about looking at my own actions and exploring my own thoughts: all day and throughout the day. I question and argue everything in my mind throughout the day constantly. It is with this tool that I have been able to dissect each thought that has influenced my behavior. It is through this rigorous analyzing of dilemmas that I have gotten peace of mind, and the instructions were outlined in this book.

Solving dilemmas was something another Ancient Greek philosopher, one who Plato gives credit of teaching Socrates the art of the dialectic did as well: Parmenides. Parmenides is quoted with saying: "There is nothing that is true, that is at some point untrue, nothing absolute that is also relative." For Parmenides, the Law of Contradiction was the only true truth. The Law of Contradiction means there can't be any truth, empirical or otherwise, which contradicts another. There are no such things as paradoxes. Parmenides and Heraclitus approached the world from two opposing views. Heraclitus thought that all we have are our senses, and Parmenides thought the physical world of the senses was some type of illusion. Parmenides claimed that all we have is the now; therefore, there is no such thing as motion, and the empirical world always contradicts itself through relativity and duality; so, the empirical world is more of an illusion.

Parmenides believed in the fact of Absolute Being. Absolute Being is the only thing that there is, and Absolute Being cannot be made of anything else, and cannot be a combination of Being and non-Being; therefore, the empirical world of motion is an illusion because anything that is moving is constantly changing, and the only thing that exists is Being, which is Absolute and does not change; therefore, the empirical world is nothing but our ignorant illusion.

Zeno, who was a student of Parmenides, said: "an arrow in flight is always in the now, in an equal place and motionless." It was with this philosophical argument that the Eleatic philosophy proved that the only thing there is, is Being in this very moment; therefore, there is no such thing as change and motion. What is real is perfect and immutable. When one takes a picture of an arrow in flight it is represented in that moment as perfectly still. All of this has gotten me to ask the question of: "what is?," and explore the empirical world and its paradoxes that Heraclitus lived by and Parmenides rejected.

Even my existence I take as a paradox, for I questioned that the first time at the age of Fourteen. I struggled even in childhood with the question: is any part even real because if everything is cause and effect what could have ever brought about that first cause?

Aristotle agreed this empirical world is true and noticed it was always in motion. Aristotle needed a justification for that first "cause" that got everything to move. Aristotle tried to justify the first cause as the "Unmoved-Mover," but that is nothing but a semantical justification through language relativity. Aristotle was justifying qualities of contradiction to an individual. Language relativity is what some scientists do in the modern day when they are suck with quantum physics or other sciences, they just say, "that is the quantum particle's nature: wave-particle duality." When it comes to light and matter, these scientists still can't solve the mathematical explanation with how quantum particles behave as a wave when looked at indirectly or as a particle when looked at directly! It is a paradox some like to justify through semantics by just using the word "nature" just like Aristotle did with "Unmoved-Mover!"

Ever since I was a little kid, and my old brother Isaac explained to me that the Earth revolves around the Sun, I have always taken "reality" as truly fascinating. "Reality" has done nothing but always encourage me to fantasize. That is one of my earliest memories I still hold to this day: looking up at the sky, thinking and about the sun and the earth; looking for a reason and a purpose in my existence and everything else as well.

Parmenides proves existence with logic, for he says: "of impossibility there could be neither knowledge, for non-being is neither realized nor expressed." It is this statement that proves my own existence and that of God. How can something come from nothing? God was and always will be. I believe that we are just a part of It. I hold myself to a conscious "choice," so I "chose" to believe that there is a God that is One. It is made up of all things and leaves nothing out: My relative term for my God is the Heraclitean Logos. This concept is also found in Hinduism.

Heraclitus believed in the Logos, and that to find the answers of the Logos one needed to look inwards. Heraclitus says: "you can never in all your goings finds the ends of the soul, though you traveled every path, so deep are its meaning." Everything is a part of one; so, to find all answers, one needs to look inward. This is what it means to continue to look at oneself. To explore one's intentions and question one's perception. My perception has been wrong many, many times. In this life, I will never stop looking within. Lots of the conclusions I have come to, I have found by looking within as well. When I can empty my mind completely, which happens every once in a while, through the way I meditate in my chapter on ADHD, I do look off into infinity just like Heraclitus says! That Truth is there for us all!

My perception used to tell me that I was the focus of everyone else's thoughts. I was judged by every person that came across my path. They all hated me; for that I was going to make sure that each one paid. I was angry and unable to see the cause for my anger. Most people took me as the angriest person they'd ever met; the funny thing was that all I wanted was love, yet I was too scared to trust anyone. It got me to ask myself: If all I want is love and acceptance then why can't I treat everyone with love and acceptance? I still work on this daily, but it is amazing to the answers of each one of all our actions is in the prayer of Saint Francis, which was the conclusion to my anger in my first book: *A Vicious Cycle*.

Just like Ralf Waldo Emerson writes about, love is the greatest teacher. It is only because of love and acceptance that I have found any happiness. I had many people that were willing to love me until I could love myself. It was through the love of others that I was able to start looking inward and analyzing my own mind which dictated my malevolent actions. For too much of my life all I could do is see what was wrong with everything. That everything started with myself, for I was so selfish as to think I was the worst of all people. I had had a traumatic childhood and suffered lots of psychological issues because of it. It was all traumas from other people's action; I was even diagnosed with PTSD because of it. Today I do believe in cause and effect; it has helped me find a reason for why all people, including myself, do what they do. That answer to why everything is the way it is, is the *Law of Karma*, or causality, or cause and effect, or Newtons' *Law of Reciprocity*. They are all the same thing: for every action there is an opposite and equal reaction, and I reward and punish myself through my own actions. God does not punish in Karma. We punish ourselves, and we either learn or we continue to suffer.

Because I have my reasons for why the things they are, I have the reason other people do what they do too, when I have their reason, I have understanding for them. When I have understanding for them, I can forgive them and be free of the burdensome hatred. I can be free of hate especially when I can pause, which meditation is the key to that for someone like me who has exactly zero impulse control neurologically! The Doctor who gave me the results of the neurological testing from UCSF was terrified when she told me: "you have no impulse control!"

When I am free of the hatred, there is nothing left for me but peace. To me peace is synonymous with happiness. When I have a clear and peaceful mind it is because I have learned the secrets to abating the conflict between my ears, for that is where all my difficulties lie. I showed in in *Pseudo-Laws and Pseudo-Morals* there is no need to hate anyone, which led to my peace. It is something I struggle with, especially in the moment, but when I can pause and reflect, which I do every morning in silent meditation for forty-five minutes and can find a solution to my behavior and unhappiness.

There is another valuable lesson that has brought me peace, and it has been whispered from Heraclitus as well. Heraclitus said: "You can never step in the same river twice." To me this is a valuable lesson, for it tells me that things are always changing. This is synonymous with *Law of Karma* too. Everything is constantly changing. The water is always flowing down stream. The river is in constant motion; in fact, everything is in a constant state of change. As I stated Heraclitus and Parmenides approached reality from the exact opposite way, but it was this quote that has taught me that I either change with things or I repeat my behavior over and suffer.

With Heraclitus, the empirical universe is in a constant state of creation and destruction, which I see everywhere! It is with the Big Bang and the Big Crunch! It is with the stars and super nova explosions that destroy stars and create solar systems like ours! Outer space itself is full of empty space where quantum particles like a proton and an anti-proton are constantly coming out of nothing, swinging around each other, then coming back together and alienating back to nothing! It is with the four seasons, which is nothing but where our planet is based on the orbit of our own star! I see this in all life as well! It is in human life as well! There was a picture of a pregnant lady on a stretcher in the war zone in Ukraine, so there is creation and destruction within creation and destruction! Everything in the empirical world is nothing but temporary!

With humanity it is how we all are born, mature, then procreate, get old, and die ourselves! That is the aging processes! Heraclitus was the first of the empiricists in the Ancient Western World and we are still in his empirical universe to this day! Relativity and duality, which is in a constant state of creation and destruction! This is shown with paradoxes everywhere!

I was walking by a bar onetime, and I hear a lady say she was a scientist to a group of people.

I stopped, turned around, and butted in to ask, "A Scientist? Of what kind?"

She responded, "Aging."

That is when I looked directly into her eyes and asked, "You mean that ten our every eleven cells in our bodies is bacteria? So, each or our bodies in over 90% bacteria, and almost every cell in our bodies is replaced every seven years including all the human cells?"

She was in shock that I knew anything about it and responded, "Yeah?!?"

That is when I point directly at her, staring right into her eyes and shouted, "Have you ever thought of asking who or what you truly are?!?"

Everyone in the whole group outside the bar busted up into laughter! Half started to walk into the bar, and she was giving a nervous laugh as she started to walk towards the street away from the crowd.

As they were all breaking up, I shouted a quote from a Vedantin Nisargadatta Maharaj that I made sure they could all hear especially her, "The body is made of food! The mind is made of thought! See them as they are! Non-identity when natural and spontaneous is liberation! You need not know what you are! Enough to know what you are not! What you are you will never know, for every realization gives new dimensions to conquer!"

I freaked them all out by questioning their reality! Even that scientist who I guess never gave much of a thought to who or what she truly was! She hopped in the car with her girlfriend that was at the street corner and sped away quickly! So, I guess the Doctors answer to that question was: No!

I see this creation and destruction everywhere just like the Ancients did, and it is only by looking within that I get to truly discover who I am as well, which I believe anyone can do with awareness, and the best way to develop awareness is through meditation, and today I am constantly working on not take myself as either my body or my mind. I take myself as just nothing but that Pure Consciousness that it talks about in the *Vedas*, which influenced the Ancient Greeks directly. It is this Pure Consciousness that I was trying to get the scientist to acknowledge what she truly was because her whole body has been replaced at least 7 times herself just by looking at her! She definitely did not look any younger than 50 herself to me! Yet, every cell in all our bodies is dying over and over, and we take ourselves as these bodies, which these ancient scriptures the *Vedas* points out we are not!

Finding out what I truly am and looking within is what gotten me to practice Vedanta today. Vedanta is a modern-day Neoplatonism, and Plato got all his inspiration from the pre-Socratics like Heraclitus and Parmenides especially. Vedanta is what Nisargadatta Maharaj practices and was a modern day guru. All the different forms of Hinduism I have explored go very well with modern science too, just like Neoplatonism, and what I have come to believe is religion and science are only mutually exclusive if someone is a fundamentalist. I take most religions as nothing but simple logic and common sense as long as one does not want to take their scriptures literally, and no matter who we are, we all have truths in what we believe, but no one has all the empirical truths in their mental cognition.

To me such concepts as *Original Sin* are nothing but a logical argument as long as one does not take it literally. The *Book of Genesis*, to me is not saying we are all inbreed descendants from two people, and the only reason anyone has dark skin is because they are offsprings of Cain. I heard an African American male make that argument in that Biological Anthropology course I took at CCSF. Nothing made me more uncomfortable than hearing someone in the year 2016 say, "the only reason anyone has dark sink is because Cain killed his broth Able." I was in shock, just like everyone else in the class! The teacher just politely changed the topic. I think even he knew he wouldn't win that one! That boy didn't stay long in that class anyways!

Original Sin to me just means this: we ate the fruit from the *Tree of Knowledge*. It does not mean there is a piece of fruit with a tree. Why did we eat the this "forbidden fruit?" Because fruit tastes sweet. All life is controlled by its desires. That is why Adam ate it after Eve because he had desire for her too, but knowledge feels good! Just like sugar tastes good! So, it means we rose from nature, and what separates us from nature and causes every problem nature does not have is our intellect! Heraclitus made the same argument when he said the nature of man is evil because we can rationalize. *Original Sin* is both a blessing and a curse!

We can drive cars. Discover lifesaving medications and treatments. Fly to outer space and land on the moon, but our intellect also is what has causes things like global warming and nuclear bombs! Intelligence is both a blessing and a curse because it causes us so many difficulties and happiness, but we take the *Bible* literally it is ridiculous! If the *Bible* is taken as an allegory, then there is lots of logic and common sense within those scriptures. Sure, some are outdated. We should no longer be practicing polygamy, which is all throughout the *Bible*, but there are universal truths in all religions that lead to nothing but simple logic and common sense like *Original Sin*, which Heraclitus came to that same conclusion.

Heraclitus also believed that fire was the monad, or the quantum particle which makes up all everything. This is quite synonymous with modern science and an Einsteinian universe where everything is made out of energy because all fire is, is the release of energy through the rearranging of electrons. Heraclitus could tell everything was just this "energy," just like Einstein proved in the *Special Theory of Relativity*, and in Chapter VI Verse 41 in the Hindu Scripture: *The Essence of Yogavasistha* it shows how everything is made of energy too: "It is the energy of Consciousness in his bodies (physical, mental, ect), as well as the motionless (or potential) energy in a stone. It is also the energy of vibration in the winds and the energy of motion in the waters." This is a Hindu scripture that goes every well with the special theory of E=MC2! Everything is nothing but energy! Even in these ancient scriptures, and this energy is nothing but Consciousness, which goes extremely well to justify how all quantum particles behave differently depending on just how they are observed! How else would an electron, or proton, or any other quantum particle know it is being looked at directly or indirectly? Quantum particles behave as particles when they are looked at directly and behave as waves when they are looked at indirectly as I have stated all throughout this essay! We have no way of explaining this with *Law of Contradiction* like I said, if everything is nothing but this Energy Consciousness that would explain the particles behavior as well!

Everything being nothing but Consciousness also goes ever well with who and what we all truly are, which is what I was pointing out to the scientists I confronted outside the bar who could not answer! When we can realize what we truly are: not this body or mind but, as is stated in the *Rgveda*: "the True Self Itself is that Pure Consciousness. That which nothing can be known in any way, and the same True Self Pure Consciousness is not different form the Ultimate Principal Brahman. Brahman is the only reality, since it is untinged by difference, the mark of ignorance, and the one thing that cannot be improved upon." To realize that everything is nothing, but this Pure Consciousness is the awakening I am striving for!

This Pure Consciousness is something that goes very well with the concepts of a non-dual reality in an empirical world of duality. As it stated in that quote from the *Rgveda*: "of which nothing can be known in anyway," for as I pointed out everything has it opposite that can be part of our senses. Well, modern science still can't even prove what makes us conscious, but we all have our experience that validates this one apodictic quality: "Existence!" I have gotten to this state a couple times in deep meditation when I can drop my body and mind and just focus that Being that is all there truly is! That Absolute Being is an experience I stive for daily that was laid out in my chapter on ADHD and is my main mental exercise: "Not being my body or my mind, but just Consciousness!" It is an experience I believe we can all get to over and over with enough dedication and practice, and that is why it is shown to us in Chapter 6 of the *Bhagavad-Gita*!

So, which one was right Parmenides or Heraclitus? Is everything perfect Being, or is this universe in a constant state of change? Heraclitus believed in these paradoxes. Heraclitus thought "knowledge only defines what is not" like Plato writes in the end of the *Theaetetus*. There was a paradox in everything, and as I proved to that Dr of Anthropology, every answer is Western Science just leads to more questions. Even Socrates thought they both had truth, for he looked into himself to find his answers, and explored the truth with the dialectic from Parmenides. I think both solutions right as well, for the contradiction of truth is not just in Being and motion but in all physical phenomena. I love the ending of Plato's *Parmenides* the most, and it is how I live my life, for it points out how there is an a-symmetry between contradiction and paradoxes when it come to the empirical world. Because the empirical world is always in flux it is "illusory." Not a complete illusion, but this empirical illusory world is this where the solutions to my insanity have been solved when I respond to my pain and learn. It is in this empirical world that I relate all modern scientific theory to mysticism and find the answers to what I truly need through reflection: "Thy self."

Einstein proved with the electromagnetic effect that light behaves as both a continuous wave and an individual particle, and this has been verified in all quantum particles. Einstein later rejected his own theory that he won the *Nobel Prize* for because he did not like paradoxes and it violated his concept of God, but the one thing quantum physics has truly verified was the skeptics of Ancient Greece and India because the quantum world is nothing but paradoxes! Quantum gravity is a paradox, and everyone took Einstein as even crazy for trying to solve! We cannot even explain how anything came together after the Big Bang because the electromagnetic effect and gravity work in opposite directions, and the electro-magnetitic effect is 1/1040 power stronger than gravity! Gravity does not exist on a quantum level! Quantum particles push each other away is they are the same charge! So, nothing should have ever come together in the first place after the Big Bang!

Another paradox with gravity, which Einstein's *General Theory of Relativity* is our best answer for that, yet one would have to ask themselves: if gravity is such a universal force, then why are the galaxies not only expanding, but at an accelerated rate? The farther the galaxy is away from us, the faster it is moving away from us. This is shown to us by measuring the wavelength of light from the different galaxies. Gravity should be slowing everything down, not increasing an expansion which is what seems to be happening if light does not change speed like Einstein says it does not!

This expansion of our space at an accelerated rate is called *Dark Energy*, and according to Einstein the speed of light remains constant at 299,792,485 meters a second. That speed cannot very according to Einstein. The only that will change is the wavelength. If a star is moving closer to us, or a galaxy, or even someone running towards me with a flashlight, the wavelength with shorten, but that speed remains constant according to Einstein. If it is moving away from us the wavelength will get longer. This is unlike any other object and is what make the speed of light the only universal measuring sick we have that we can use across the whole universe! But our universe is expanding at an accelerated rate! Which we currently cannot explain!

We also need *Dark Matter* to keep all out galaxies rotating at the speeds they are using Einstein's *General Theory of Relativity*, which means the visible universe is only 4% of the matter that is in the universe! Neither *Dark Energy* nor *Dark Matter* has been proven! They are all just theories and assumptions to justify and explain empirical phenomena that we have no explanation for! All empirical truth has contradictions just like Plato wrote in the *Parmenides* and *Theaetetus*, and all we all do, whether we are conscious of it or not, is take what our minds tells us to. I would argue most of us just ignore rest unconciously. I have found lots of doctors in philosophy and other sciences do this because not too many of us like to realize how uncertain this empirical world truly is for themselves either! We all want things to believe in!

Think of how many people believe in the atom without understanding the math or principles behind it. Most people don't know what the Pauli Exclusion Principle is, or how there are different flavors of quarks and different masses of leptons. I am familiar with those terms, yet I don't understand the entire math behind all of them. That doesn't stop me from believing in the atom. Because I take God as everything it has shown me that science and religion have three things in common: They both give me a reason, they both give me an explanation, and they both require faith! All those theories I mentioned above require faith!

Modern science stems from one place: Ancient Greek Mythology. Sure, taken literally it is quite crazy, but there are lots of truths in all religions. Even Ancient Greek Mythology. Each Greek God was nothing but an empirical phenomenon of this universe and is just meant to explain things! They all had their exaggerated human character defects that caused all kinds of troubles as well, but they were allegories and parables just like any scripture, which means they were just like the *Bible*. We are all looking for the same thing in this life. We all want a reason, explanation, and purpose for being here, and we all use faith to achieve those if we are just using science and are atheist or we are religious thesis!

Modern science is always making assumptions in order to come up with new theories to explain phenomena just like *Dark Energy* and *Dark Matter*. We make assumptions, then we measure the consequences of those assumptions through empirical testing. Those assumptions are impossible to prove, like with the *Theory of Relativity*. Einstein made the assumption that the speed of light remains constant for all observers. That is an impossible assumption to prove. We would need to trace a photon of light from one end or our Universe to another and make sure that it never varied in speed! That is an obvious test that cannot be performed! Einstein made that assumption, then he measured the consequences of that assumption! So, Einstein used faith too! But it was that specific assumption that allowed for the best theory we have of gravity and motion that still holds to this day, and that assumption is nothing but an article of faith!

One way to explain that accelerated expansion of the universe I read once was that the speed of light doesn't remain constant but loses energy over extremely long distances. Like billions and billions of light-years. This would turn the *Theory of Relativity* on its' head! My point is none of us truly know! All we have is speculation when it comes to the empirical world, and life requires faith whether you believe in God or not. I don't deny the empirical world because my mind only develops by interacting with it, but Modern Science is always wrong! Especially if they do not acknowledge the paradoxes everywhere in an empirical world of relativity and duality! It is also impossible to prove that the Speed of Light remains constant like Einstein says! It is an assumption! Motion is relative means that perspective it relative, along with an individual truth, and once again with duality: everything existing having its opposites? All this shows me is life is always about learning, and learning is always about constantly admitting the mistakes in our beliefs so we can always get to better answers, which is what modern science is all about! Overthrowing one theory for another!

It is important to acknowledge that even when I take an experience as an empirical fact, I am still using faith. I have had times in my life where I saw and heard things that were not there. I have even talked to things that I now know weren't there. This is why I have had reasons to doubt, not just my senses, but my rational mind as well. As I said it is not doing the same thing over and over and expecting a different result, but when I cannot question my sanity, or the conclusions my mind comes to, is where my insanity lies, and looking throughout world history and even the current news it seems to me that is the cause with the rest of the world too!

Not too many of us like to admit we are wrong, but with this doubt I have had the clarity to see that I need faith, and we all use faith. Faith has showed me what to take as a subjective reality: Faith and my innate perception, for that is all anyone has. Most people have a hard time questioning themselves. I have also seen myself that it is the really crazy people that can't question their own sanity as I pointed out in my chapter on Schizophrenia. Most "sane" people I have talked to have no ability to question their sanity either; so, does this mean that most people aren't any different than a lunatic because we all believe things that are not true? So, what truly is the difference between a false belief and a delusion, especially if someone has no ability to question themselves?

With all of my insanity it is my doubt that has saved me. Only when I questioned my own reality was I able to find any answers. My eyes and ears have led me astray before, and how does anyone truly know if something is happening to them at this very moment? Everyone needs to be able to question themselves and their sanity!

There is someone I know who is struggling with sobriety. It is impossible for him to acknowledge that there is even such a thing as faith. He is someone who was raised by Jehovah's Witnesses, and it made him hate everything about religion, and he refuses to see any truth in the aspects of God. He even tells me Einstein's theories are Laws.

I pointed out to this man that Einstein spent the second half of his life trying to reconcile the *Electromagnetic Effect* and *General Relativity* and he couldn't. Gravity is a paradox on a quantum level as I stated before, and everyone took Einstein as even crazy for trying to reconcile it. It was Wolfgang Pauli said, "That is a solution that is better left up to God!" I suggested to a professor on his blog that I took a graduate class on relativity from that I read an article once that the universe isn't expanding, at least at accelerated rates, but that light is retarded over long distances, which would explain the expansion of the universe, so there would be no need for *Dark Energy*. I also suggested my own theory that maybe this retardation of light, and the loss of light's energy over billions of lightyears, could be tied to quantum gravity somehow? That these photons of light not remaining constant, but slowly losing energy and speed over billions and billions of lightyears could be tied to the quantification of gravity because light being a constant speed was the thing Einstein was unwilling to give up in order to unite the *Electromagnetic Effect* and the *General Theory of Relativity*! That loss of energy over extremely long distances might be a way to reconcile the repulsion of like against like on quantum levels!

That just seemed to freak the professor out that I gave him a possible solution to the quantification of gravity, but this man, who is struggling to get sober, wants something to believe in just like the people he condemns who raised him as a child, so he believes in the greatness of Einstein, who was truly great! Yet, he refuses to acknowledge the fact that he is using faith constantly! He can't even do a geometrical tensor, which is necessary to understand the *General Theory of Relativity*, yet he calls Einstein's Theories a Laws. That is also why this ex-Jehovah's Witness calls it a Law because he does not understand it! It is nothing but faith for him too! Yet, he refuses to acknowledge the word faith!

I had the same problem that man had for years! I was surrounded by fundamentalists in Provo Utah, who all thought they were doing the right thing. These Fundamentalists thinking that they were doing the right thing just made my life a living Hell! I had been sent to that school Discovery Academy because I was abused and flipped out because of that abuse. The fundamentalist beliefs just made me a million times worse than I already was, and every kid I have talked to from the place all told me the same thing! Not that they thought those fundamentalists were doing what they thought was right, but that Discovery Academy only made them much, much worse!

Those kids at Discovery Academy all also told me that Dr had them on all the wrong medications with the wrong diagnoses too! It was not just me! So, I understood what this guy I know, who was brought up by Jehovah's Witnesses, went through in one way or another. Discovery Academy just made me hate God more than anything because none of us kids who were locked up there were Mormon except one. We were all being abused with isolation and bad medical treatment, and they would not stop trying to convert all of us at the same time! We all hated anything to do with that Church except one student who converted. His last name was Jones, so we all called him Jesus Jones!

But, if that guy who was raised by the Jehovah's Witnesses understood anything about Einstein, all Einstein's theories would still be a theories that needs to be proven false, just like all other theories! His faith is in science, just like the assumption that Einstein made about the speed of light being constant! Science using faith was something my first philosophy professor William Graves taught me. That man who can't stay sober, is sure he has all the answers, and I would say to him if he truly did, he'd be both happy and sober, and he is not. He has no ability to admit he does not know, and that is what kept me from learning any truth for a big part of my life. He is just as narrow minded as the people who he condemns just like I was, and just like so many of us are. It is what drove me so nuts my whole drug and alcohol abuse too! I could not admit I did not have the answers and I could barely read!

When it comes to truth of the empirical world all I have is conjecture. That is all anyone has: the paradox of "choice" based on the strict enforcement of experience. First, I was an atheist, then an agnostic, and now I found something that I can believe in. Something that has all the answers. It shows me that all of my answers are either in front of or within me, as long as I have an open mind, which means I can always be wrong about everything except "I Am," and it has led to happiness. When I first defined God, I called it: "Everything I Did

Not Know and Did Not Understand." This way I could learn. I would argue that because of what I just proved above, and all throughout this book, that is a provable definition of God! Those words: "I Don't Know" has turned into everything including myself; "I Don't Know" are the only words that are able to honestly answer every question that is presented in front of each one of us and being able to answer every question is something only God can do. I met a professor who had a PhD in theology who said my definition was very Socratic.

My life is all about admitting when I do not know just as Socrates taught: "The only thing I know, is I know nothing." The whole point is none of us know much in this world of relativity and duality because of paradox after paradox after paradox! This is because everything being in constant change through creation and destruction: Karma, but what guides me is perfect and immutable within me. My solution is staying in the moment, and as I heard a wise man say once "there is infinite time in the present moment." It is also why I have meditated every day for forty-five minutes for the past six years. It got me to see just the other day that the *Law of Karma* and the *Theory of Evolution* both tells me the same thing in silent meditation: everything is constantly changing and I either learn or I suffer. If I want this empirical world to be perfect, I just need to acknowledge it is nothing but my perfect teacher! I need an absolute radical acceptance that I just need to change for the better! It does not matter what anyone else does! I am still working on this idea to this day because that is all it is for me! A perfect ideal, just like all dogma that is not taken literally! I need to change to adapt to it or I suffer. I believe this is the essence of all our plights that each of us are in the center of in my metaphysical theory!

Perfect ideals and directions of the objective truth is what we should all always strive for, which means we just make progress. I have found happiness in my life by exploring answers, looking for the truth of the empirical world, and acknowledging my ignorance. It has all been laid in front of us by the Ancients and taught to us by each experience we have been through. I also believe it is a universal truth within us all!

To me it is in the lessons of life that we all can find happiness, and that is why discord is a necessity. It is the pain of our consequences, and learning from that pain, that will lead us all to happiness. That pain has taught me a provable definition of God, the words "I Don't Know," but if you want awareness without being beaten into it, then just sit in silence and meditate. I have found the best way in my chapter on ADHD, and it is the corner stone of getting off all of my psych medications. Remember, awareness is the greatest virtue because the recognition of a problem is the first step in anything. Without awareness nothing changes for the better, and you can either be beaten into it, or seek it on a daily basis through silent meditation. Someone told me once that "I pray for a lower tolerance of pain because that is the only reason I change for the better." I still use that as my guiding prayer to this day.

So, it is important to note that God is provable depending on how you define it! This is what got me into yoga. The God of the *Rgveda* is also a provable definition of God! It is nothing but Consciousness, and every experience I have validates one thing over and over no matter what that experience is: I am conscious! All of your experiences validate that you are conscious. What those experiences truly are, are all subject to doubt, but each and every single one of them proves existence through Consciousness! As Nisargadatta Maharaj says in the book *I Am That*, "as every taste of salt pervades the great ocean, and every drop of seawater carries the same flavor, so every experience gives me the touch of reality. The ever-fresh realization of my own being." If one sits in silence and focuses just on the words "I am," they can get to the point where they can slowly stop thinking, and when you are able to drop your mind completely, you can experience the perfection within you which is Simple, Immutable, Perfect, Complete, but besides those descriptions is Ineffable. It is ineffable because it is non-dual. It is something they say that can only be experienced through the thinning of the mind which is laid out in ancient scriptures.

But is there a God, and does this life have any mean? These are questions, like Parmenides said, are truly only answered in one place: "everyone runs away from death; therefore, they run away from the truth." It is only in death that I truly find out if this life means anything or not. If I die and I exist, then there is a reason and a purpose to this existence. If I die and I don't, then that is my answer, but as of now having a provable definition of God that is Socratic and scientific has led to a happy life, and so does the *Vedas*.

I am someone who has tried killing myself more times than I can count, and today because of my belief system, I am a very happy person who is seeking answers. I am also off all psych medications today because of this book and my belief system. I have been on almost every psych medication in the PDR at one time of my life too. If I have to take them again I will, but I am grateful to be off all thought retarding medications for psych issues and epilepsy. I have found happiness, not by getting everything I want, but by looking within myself today and finding God!

Remember God is just a word, and there is relativity in langue as well. The same words mean different things to different people. Some people take God as a white male in the sky. I don't hold to that literal interpretation, for that interpretation is more making God in our image, not God making us in its. That definition just leads to conflict and insanity to me. In this essay, I prove God in two ways: "I don't know" and "Consciousness."

"Consciousness" is how all the mystics of all religions define God. It is in the Jewish scripture the *Kabbala*. Ibn al-Arabi defined God this way and Sufi mysticism, which is nothing but a combination of Hinduism and Islamic beliefs. Something lot of modern-day Buddhists refuse to acknowledge is the Buddha was nothing but a Hindu. All this concepts such and pleasure and pain, selfish desires being the main cause of all the suffering, and Atman and Brahman are all Vedic concepts that come out of the *Vedas*. The Buddhists and the Hindus are talking about the same thing. One calls it God the other says it is everything and all powerful but refuses to use the word God because on the topic the Buddha remained silent, but the Buddha was not a nihilist. When someone mentioned the term God, the Buddha just did say anything, but they are both Hinduism and Buddhism are talking about the same thing, which is nothing but langue relativity when one says it is all powerful but there is no such thing as God, and the other call it God, and they both define it as Consciousness.

The term Buddha is all throughout the *Bhagavad-Gita*, which is dated somewhere in the second millennium BCE or before, some say the *Gita* is even as early as the Bronze Age! The Buddha did not come until 5th or 6th century BCE. Buddha is just a Sanskrit word for anyone who is awake! Anyone who has touched and gotten in contact with the "Consciousness" that is everything and within us all! They are talking about the same thing.

Searching for this "Consciousness" is what has led to my happiness, and I have faith this happiness is within us all! It is Sat-Chit-Ananda, or Being-Consciousness-Bliss, as it teaches in Vedanta, and that happiness is a Non-Dual Being-Happiness that I believe is within all of us, it is a Happiness that can be kept in any situation because it is a Happiness that has no opposite, and can be tapped into with unrelentless daily effort of single pointed concentration meditation (Trataka) with the cultivated ability to drop one's mind completely! It is there for anyone to experience, which is the proof we all need! Just be willing to learn and question everything! Look for your certainty in only one thing: I Am! Not a literal interpretation of a scripture because that is nothing but fear! Fundamentalism is about the impossible: certainty in an uncertain world! We find certainty in one place only: Existence!

WORKS CITED

Chapter 2: A Glimmer of Hope

Ellison, Ralph, *Invisible Man*, The New American Library Inc., New York, ©1952

Plotinus, Translated by Taylor, Tomas, *An Essay on the Beautiful*, London, ©1917

Plotinus, Translated by Stephen MacKenna, *The Enneads*, Penguin Books, ©1991

Robin, Leon, *Greek Thought, and the Origins of the Scientific Spirit* Routledge, ©1998

Chapter 3: Pseudo-Laws and Pseudo-Morals

Bible, King James

Aquinas, Thomas, Edited Introduction by Baumgarth, William P., and Regan, Richard J. *On Law, Morality, and Politics*, Hackett Publishing Company ©1988

I Am That, Talks with Sri Nisargadatta Maharaj, ©1973 by Nisargadatta Maharaj

Greek Thought and the Origins of the Scientific Spirit, Robin, Leon Routledge, ©1998

The Conceptual Risks of Risk Assessment, K.S. Shrader-Frechette IEEE Technology and Society Magazine, ©1986 June 1986

The Real Risks of Risk-Cost-Benefit Analysis, K.S. Shrader-Frechette Technology In Society Vol. 7 pp 399 to 409 ©1986

Michigan Vs. EPA, Leading Case Study Harvard Law Review, Case 153 S. Ct. 2699, 129 ©2015, Harv. L. Rev 311, 11/10/15

Roe vs Wade, (1973) The United States Supreme Court, Jane Roe, et al., Appellants, Vs Henry Wade, 93 S. Ct 705, *No. 70-18*, Argued: December 13th 1971, Reargued October 11th 1972, Decided January 22nd 1973, Rehearing Denied February 26th 1973, Overturned June 24th 2022

MATAL, INTERIM DIRECTOR, UNITED STATES PATENT AND TRADEMARK OFFICE v. TAM, United States Supreme Court, The Supreme Court Of the United States, Matal Vs. Tam, Joseph Matal, Interim Director, United States Patent and Trade Mark Office, Petitioner, vs Simon Shioa Tam, No. 15-1293, Argued Jan 18th 2016/ Decided Jun 19th 2017

Chapter 4: The Power of Inaction

UCSF Neurological Evaluation: Garcia, Paul MD
Evaluation done by: Kopald, Brandon E. Psy.D., ABPP-CN 09-14-2017

Gosh, Shyam *Rgveda for the Layman,* Munshiram Monoharlal Publishing ©2014

Freud, Sigmund Translated by Brill, A.A., *The Sigmund Freud Collection* ©2016 Sigmund Freud

I Am That, Talks with Sri Nisargadatta Maharaj, ©1973 by Nisargadatta Maharaj

Chapter 7: Overcoming Depression

Shakespeare, William, *The Tragedy of Hamlet, Prince of Denmark,* ©1604

Chapter 8: Overcoming Schizophrenia and Bipolar

Physic World, *Dark Matter and Energy,* ©01/18/2017 https://physicsworld.com/a/dark-energy-emerges-when-energy-conservation-is-violated/

Reichenbach, Hans, Translated by Reichenbach, Maria and Freund John, *The Philosophy of Space and Time,* New York ©1958

Sellars, Wilfred, *Empiricism and Philosophy of the Mind,* Harvard University Press, Cambridge Massachusetts. London, England, ©1997

Azadpur, Mohammad, *Knowing the Unknown, and Avicennian Perspective of Sellarian Empiricism*

Landy, David, *A Recent Scholarship on Hume's Theory of Mental Representation*

Nasar, Sylvia, *A Beautiful Mind, The Life of Mathematical Genius and Nobel Laureate John Nash,* Simon & Schuster Paperbacks, New York, London, Toronto, Sydney

Descartes, Rene, *Meditations on the First Philosophy,* ©2013, Seedbox Press

Brandom, Robert B., *Articulating Reasons, An Introduction to Inferentialism*, ©2000, Harvard University Press Cambridge, Massachusetts, London England

Marx, Karl and Engels, Fredrick *On Religion*, ©1883 Dover Publications, New York

WiseGeek: https://www.wisegeek.com/of-all-that-we-see-how-much-can-the-brain-process.htm

St. Dionysius the Areopagite, Translated by John Parker, *The Works of Dionysius the Areopagite*

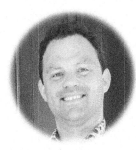 **JUSTIN WITTE** is an author, life coach and motivational speaker. He's worked as a tutor and speaks at nonprofits helping people who struggle with mental illness and other disabilities. Justin speaks from his experience with eight different physical and mental disorders, along with addiction issues. Justin, originally from Oregon, lives in San Francisco and is currently pursuing a Master's in Philosophy at San Francisco State University. This collection of poetry and essays is his second book.

COLOPHON

The text of *The Shadowed Soul* is set in Adobe Garamond Pro. Created in the 16th century by Claude Garamond, a Parisian engraver, the typeface has elegant glyphs (e.g. the ff & *ff*), old-style numerical forms, and is considered a legibility classic for book text. The italic forms were created by Robert Granjon during the same period. In 1989 Robert Slimback, an Adobe type designer, adapted Garamond for digital use.

The chapter titles are set in Semplicita Pro which is a modern adaptation of Alessandro Butti's typeface, *Semplicità*, created in the 1930s for the Nebiolo type foundry.

Text for the author's biography and back cover of the book is set in Neutraface. It's geometric sans-serif forms were designed for digital use by Christian Schwartz for House Industries. Neutraface derives its name and inspiration from the work of architect Richard Neutra. Dion Neutra, his son and former partner, helped develop the typeface.